D1460019

THE SUPER
SIMPLE
HCG DIET

KATHLEEN BARNES

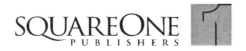

SQUAREONE
PUBLISHERS

Cover Designer: Jeannie Tudor
Editor: Michael Weatherhead
Typesetter: Terry Wiscovitch

The information and advice contained in this book are based upon the research and the personal and professional experiences of the author. They are not intended as a substitute for consulting with a health care professional. The publisher and author are not responsible for any adverse effects or consequences resulting from the use of any of the suggestions, preparations, or procedures discussed in this book. All matters pertaining to your physical health should be supervised by a health care professional. It is a sign of wisdom, not cowardice, to seek a second or third opinion.

The BMI Chart on page 51 appears courtesy of www.wikipedia.org.

Square One Publishers
115 Herricks Road
Garden City Park, NY 11040
(516) 535-2010 • (866) 900-BOOK
www.squareonepublishers.com

Library of Congress Cataloging-in-Publication Data

Barnes, Kathleen, 1956-
  The super simple HCG diet : the simplest and most successful way to shed excess weight / Kathleen Barnes.
    p. cm.
  Includes bibliographical references and index.
  ISBN 978-0-7570-0375-2 (alk. paper)
1. Low-calorie diet. 2. Weight loss. 3. Chorionic gonadotropins--Diet therapy. I. Title.
  RM222.2.B376 2011
  613.2'5—dc23

                                                2011023134

Printed in Canada

10   9   8   7   6   5   4   3   2   1

Contents

Foreword, vii

Introduction, 1

1. My Journey, 5

2. Simplifying the Simeons Protocols, 11

3. What You Can Eat and What You Can't, 27

4. Shots or Drops?, 41

5. When the Time Is Right, 49

6. HCG is for Men Too!, 55

7. Navigating the Potholes, 61

8. Building Self-Esteem, 75

9. Keeping the Weight Off, 81

Conclusion, 85

Calorie Counts, 87

Glycemic Index Chart, 91

Resources, 93

Diet Diary, 97

About the Author, 127

Index, 129

To my beloved Joe, proofreader, omelet maker
and cheerleader extraordinaire;
and my dear friend Dr. Hyla Cass,
physician, healer and chief encourager.

I love you both.

I couldn't have made it without
the two of you.

Foreword

I am an enthusiastic supporter of the HCG diet. At a time when two-thirds of American adults are overweight and approximately 26 percent are obese, I see the HCG diet as an innovative way to address a serious national problem. It provides hope for millions who have been unable to achieve permanent weight loss. I have witnessed easy, safe and well-proportioned long-term weight loss in scores of my patients.

The original HCG diet as formulated by Dr. Simeons nearly sixty years ago is very effective and perfectly achievable. Even with the appetite-suppressing effects of HCG, however, a 500-calorie-per-day diet may be difficult to sustain, especially for those who have more than twenty-five pounds to lose. I applaud health writer and advocate Kathleen Barnes—a longtime friend, coauthor, sometime patient, and author of *The Super Simple HCG Diet*—for her contributions to our knowledge of the HCG diet, and particularly for her thoughts on how to use the program for an extended period of time.

Kathleen broke new ground by remaining on the diet without taking the breaks recommended by Dr. Simeons. By slightly relaxing the program to 700 calories a day, she experienced regular and rapid weight loss (100 pounds in a little over eight months) while remaining energetic and committed to the process. While I generally suggest breaks after a cycle of twenty-three to forty-three days, I have had patients who, like Kathleen, successfully continued the regimen non-stop for several months, accompanied by a nutrient-rich protocol of essential vitamins and minerals.

In her version of the HCG diet, Kathleen allows additional low-glycemic-index vegetables and fruits to help vary the meal plan, and also includes soups, increasing the likelihood that you will actually follow the diet over the long-term and reach your target weight. Finally, she relates her experiences with diet "potholes," providing invaluable information that can guide you towards success.

I enthusiastically watched Kathleen's progress. She is now at least as well versed in nutrition and natural health as any licensed doctor, and probably has a greater depth of knowledge in this field than most. With *The Super Simple HCG Diet*, Kathleen Barnes makes a vital contribution to our understanding of this subject and helps bring the program into the twenty-first century. She forges a new path, and her modification to the diet is effective and well-grounded in present-day knowledge. She gives a gift to overweight people all over the world that will help them attain weight-loss success and prevent the myriad health problems that go hand in hand with obesity. I commend her, and recommend that you read and apply the wisdom of this book to your own life.

Hyla Cass, MD
Pacific Palisades, CA

Introduction

I've made a career of writing about health. I've contributed hundreds of articles to various health-related publications and worked as a natural health columnist for *Woman's World* magazine for six years. I've been an ardent advocate of natural living for my entire adult life, yet I haven't always walked my talk. While I ate a fairly healthful diet, I simply ate too much. After behaving in this manner for twenty years, I ended up 100 pounds overweight. Yikes! Thankfully, I found out about the HCG diet.

Having written for numerous health publications over the past fifteen years, as well as being the author of more than a dozen health books, I recognize a good thing when I see it. In fact, the HCG diet is more than a good thing. It is a revolutionary weight-loss method that leads to lifelong weight control, and it can eliminate America's obesity problem. With approximately two-thirds of Americans considered obese, we are at a crisis point in this country. Conventional medicine has little to offer except the admonition to "eat less and exercise more." But this advice is not enough. It is time to illuminate a real cure for this problem.

While HCG certainly seems like the magic pill you've been waiting for, this doesn't mean you can take it and eat anything you want. I want to make this clear from the beginning. The HCG diet is a rigorous low-calorie regimen. The "magic" is the fact that HCG allows you to stay on the diet for months at a time without being tempted to eat your desk, your pillow or (God forbid!) your spouse.

When I tell people about the original HCG diet, they often think it is entirely too complicated. They worry that 500 calories might not be enough for basic survival and cringe at the idea of injecting themselves with a hormone. I understand these concerns completely. The purpose of this book is to help you overcome these fears by simplifying the HCG diet. It is not hocus-pocus. It is simply a matter of being able to adhere to a low-calorie, low-carb, low-fat and low-glycemic-index meal plan. It's a tall order, but this is where HCG comes into the picture. Granted, it doesn't work for everyone, but, in my experience, HCG allowed me to maintain this strict weight-loss routine painlessly. It has helped tens of thousands of other dieters do the same.

I am not giving you medical advice in this book. I am merely sharing my journey, helping to quell your fears about the low-calorie aspect of the diet (I think 700 calories is more realistic, and I'll explain why), trying to reduce your anxiety about injections, and giving you alternatives if you don't feel you can handle the shots. Before I began the program, I needed to know as much as I could about what I was about to get myself into. As a health journalist, I know not to take information at face value. I like to dig for the real facts. Once I had the facts about the original HCG diet, I set off to use my own personal version of the weight-loss routine.

By following the diet, I discovered a number of significant considerations that were absent from the literature on the subject. This book is an attempt to provide you not only with these considerations but also with little tips and tricks that you won't find in other texts. It also answers the most common questions I've received concerning the HCG diet.

I am pleased to offer my personal experiences as a vehicle to inspire you, help you on your journey, and give you the confidence to undertake this life-changing program. I hope that you share your experience with others.

Kathleen Barnes

My Journey

I t's a fairly pathetic story that will be all too familiar to most of my readers: I pretty much managed to keep my weight under control until I hit menopause. For me, however, that phase of life had to be surgically accelerated, so I began to experience it in my early forties.

The first year, I put on about five pounds. That didn't seem too bad, but then I added another five pounds a year later and yet another five a year after that. Over the span of twenty years, in fact, I packed on 100 pounds. I looked and felt like a blimp. Even today, I find it hard to admit how much I weighed when I began my simplified version of the HCG diet. Moreover, my weight was especially embarrassing because I write books and magazine articles about natural health for a living. I certainly wasn't a good example of the healthful lifestyle I had been advocating!

Although you might suspect otherwise, my eating habits at the time were actually pretty good. I ate nutritious food. The problem was that I ate a lot of it. It seemed like the mechanism in charge of shutting off my hunger was simply broken. Every time I ate something, I'd get a craving for something else. I never counted calories, because I didn't want to, but I was most likely consuming over 3,000 calories a day. I couldn't stop eating and was told that hunger was a common menopause-related pitfall. I could try to blame the weight gain on any number of reasons—low thyroid, elevated insulin, out-of-whack brain chemistry—but, in reality, how I'd gained it didn't really matter. I was fat.

FROM DESPERATION TO HOPE

I don't know when I got to the point of desperation, but I got there. I tried every sensible and nonsensical diet around. Nothing worked. I'd stick to the diet until 4:00 P.M. (sound familiar?), at which point I'd get a raging sugar craving (dark chocolate is healthy, right?) or an irresistible urge for a big bowl of butter-drenched popcorn. Sometimes I'd want both! I was very fortunate to have avoided any of the obvious health complications associated with morbid obesity, such as diabetes, hypertension, high cholesterol, heart disease and stroke. Perhaps my generally healthful diet had helped me to do so. I continued to avoid processed foods, trans-fats, high-fructose corn syrup and most of the other baddies found in supermarket aisles, but I was still overeating and unable to find a way to lose weight that worked for me. I needed a reason to hope.

One day, I ran into my good friend Frankie Boyer while attending a conference. She looked terrific! I won't presume to estimate how much unwanted poundage she had shed, but it was an amazing transformation. That was the first time I heard about the HCG diet, and the first time I felt a glimmer of hope. Unfortunately, that hope was almost completely dashed when I realized that the HCG diet sounded too difficult for me to follow.

Inspired by research done by Dr. A.T.W. Simeons during the 1950s, the HCG diet is defined by a set of requirements that have come to be known as the Simeons Protocols, which Dr. Simeons outlines in his book *Pounds and Inches*. According to the work of Dr. Simeons, HCG—a hormone produced during pregnancy that plays a role in sustaining and protecting the growing fetus—curbs the appetite and encourages the body to burn fat rather than muscle. (See the inset "What Is HCG?" on page 12.) The Simeons Protocols recommend taking one injection of HCG, also known as *human chorionic gonadotropin*, and eating no more than 500 calories each day. In addition, those calories must come from a very limited range of foods. The diet also prohibits the use of all skin creams, moisturizers and supplements (including fish oil). Sound difficult? I thought so, too. That's why I put the idea on the back burner.

The little fairy that had pricked my consciousness with the idea, however, rose up again a few months later when I heard about a simplified version of the HCG diet that recommends a more sustainable and healthier 700-calorie-a-day meal plan along with a few other adjustments to the rigid Simeons Protocols. I was hooked. I began to believe I might actually be able to follow the diet without starving. Hope had returned.

SEALING THE DEAL

The universe works in strange ways. Just a few days after I'd heard about the 700-calorie version of the diet, I met Katherine, a woman who has spent twenty-five years in recovery from alcohol and food addiction. Part of Katherine's poignant story was her tale of meeting a beautiful woman at an Alcoholics Anonymous meeting on a beach in Hawaii. Katherine was feeling fat and dumpy at the time and was entranced by the woman's beauty and grace. Oddly, the woman approached her and, after a brief conversation, left her with a piece of advice. "Don't eat sugar or flour," she said. Katherine listened. In a few short months, she was slim and attractive, living in what she now calls a "right-sized" body. Her dedication inspired me and made me think of what I might accomplish on the HCG diet.

The final puzzle piece fell into place within a week of my encounter with Katherine. I was talking on the phone with my dear friend Dr. Hyla Cass, a holistic physician and health book author who selflessly shares sound medical advice. I mentioned all the signs I had been experiencing, which I felt were pushing me to get started on the HCG diet, and she graciously offered to guide me through the plan. She told me the results experienced by her patients on the HCG diet had been "miraculous." All of these serendipitous events sealed the deal for me. It was time. The means had been provided. I would do it.

TAKING THE LEAP

I began the HCG diet one November. Although doses of HCG are available as oral drops—a method that Dr. Cass and many happy dieters, including several friends and my daughter, assure me is as effective as the alternative—I chose to use injections of the hormone, which must be prescribed by a doctor. Eight and a half months later, I am 100 pounds lighter (though I *feel* about 1,000 pounds lighter). It was basically a smooth journey—I even took a couple of hiatuses for holidays and travel—but I wasn't a saint. Occasionally, I gave in to hunger pangs or, more likely, psychological cravings. But when I got on that scale every morning and saw how much unwanted fat I'd shed, it perked me up so much that I got right back on the plan. The fact that I've reached my goal and completed my journey is enormously satisfying. It has positively affected both my health and my self-esteem.

This book is the story of my journey. It's not a medical book. It's simply my experience. I will share with you the insights I have gained along the way, as well as a few techniques that can help you avoid some of the potholes that await you on the road to better health.

WATCH WHAT YOU THINK

One pothole I'd like to mention right now concerns the power of thought. Now, there's nothing that annoys me more than people who try to tell me how to think, but this advice is truly important. If you constantly think and talk about "losing" weight, your trusting subconscious mind, which is really nothing more than a self-centered child without powers of discrimination, begins to think you are losing a part of yourself. Of course, subconsciously, you will not want to lose any part of yourself, even if that part is killing you. By approaching your weight in this way, you may be sabotaging your chance of success.

To avoid this problem, all you need to do is adjust your perception slightly. I found it helpful to think and tell others that I was "controlling" or "reducing" my weight. It's just a little thing, but it can be immensely consequential. As my unwanted weight continues to stay off, I am reminded of what an important force for change thought truly is.

Conclusion

Now that you know a little bit about my story, the following chapter will take a closer look at the traditional HCG diet and explain ways in which you can adjust its stringent routine to make it a little more manageable. Rather than feeling intimidated and put off by a diet that seems impossible to follow, you will feel empowered and excited once you understand that my simplified version is both effective and sustainable.

2

Simplifying the Simeons Protocols

M any news outlets have reported on the HCG diet. Some stories have had positive spins, while others have been negative. In most cases, the information has been boiled down to sound bites that offer little detail and almost no science. This type of poor information can easily stop your weight-loss plan in its tracks before you even get a chance to see the amazing results the HCG diet can provide. You may decide that the diet is too difficult or just plain untrue, either of which would be tragic. To clear up the confusion, you must first explore what the HCG diet is and how it can be made simple and sustainable. Only then will you get a sense of this miracle program's true potential.

IN THE BEGINNING

Just after World War II, British physician and researcher Dr. A.T.W. Simeons began a study of overweight patients at his clinic in Rome, Italy. A few years later, in 1954, he published its startling findings, which showed that daily injections of the hormone human chorionic gonadotropin, or HCG, enabled patients to remain on a diet of only 500 calories per day. What's more, Dr. Simeons found that HCG appeared to burn fat rather than muscle mass, accelerating the body's natural fat-burning process and trimming away fat in all the crucial places. In recent years, new theories have suggested that HCG may encourage the body's master hormone gland, known as the *hypothalamus*, to reset your body's entire hormone system, known as the *endocrine system*. By hitting your "reset button," your body begins to see its reduced size as normal, creating a new default weight so that it doesn't try to regain what it has lost.

Dr. Simeons' book *Pounds and Inches* became a hit in the 1950s and briefly received wide attention. In the book, he described the methods he had used to create rapid weight loss, which are now called the Simeons Protocols. Comprising three phases, Dr. Simeons' system includes twenty-three to forty daily injections of HCG, depending on the desired amount of weight loss. Phase one begins with a two-day food binge that encourages a high intake of fatty foods in particular. For the remainder of the HCG treatments, the dieter follows phase two, which is defined by an extremely rigid 500-calorie-per-day diet. Once the injections are finished, the

What Is HCG?

Human chorionic gonadotrophin, or HCG, is a hormone that is naturally produced by a woman's body when she is pregnant. Made from the cells that form the placenta, it nourishes a fertilized egg after it is implanted in the uterine wall. It has been approved by the FDA for the treatment of both male and female infertility. Its exact mechanism in weight loss is unknown, but it seems to curb appetite and direct the body to burn fat instead of muscle.

"reset" stage starts, known as phase three. During this phase, caloric restriction is maintained for an additional three-day period, after which the dieter is permitted to increase food intake but must continue to refrain from eating sugar and starches for a full three weeks. Should the dieter wish to lose more weight, another course of the HCG diet may be undertaken after a six-week break. Additional rounds and longer breaks are followed as necessary.

The guidelines of the diet are severe and difficult to follow, not to mention unbelievably boring. They call for seven ounces of very lean meat—including beef, chicken breast, fresh white fish, lobster, crab, veal, or shrimp—to be eaten per day, half at lunch and half at dinner. The meat must be weighed raw and have all visible fat removed. In addition, only one type of vegetable is allowed at both lunch and dinner, and must be chosen from the following group: spinach, chard, chicory, beet greens, salad greens, tomatoes, celery, fennel, onions, red radishes, cucumbers, asparagus and cabbage. One breadstick and one piece of a limited selection of fruit (an apple, orange, handful of strawberries or half a grapefruit) are added to both meals.

Breakfast is generally made up of tea or coffee in any quantity you wish. But keep in mind that only one tablespoon of milk per day is allowed while on Dr. Simeons' HCG diet. Saccharin may be used a sweetener, but considering the health concerns regarding artificial sweeteners that have come to light lately, I would avoid it. In addition to coffee and tea, plain water and mineral water are allowed in unlimited quantities. Seasonings and the juice of one lemon per day are permitted for cooking, but oils, butters and dressings are not.

Finally, the Simeons Protocols prohibit all medicines, including dietary supplements; all makeup except powder, lipstick and eyebrow pencil; and all face creams and moisturizers, under the assumption that the fats in these products can upset your body's fat-burning mechanism.

WHAT SCARED ME AWAY

Wow! When I first read the Simeons Protocols, I absolutely knew there was no way I could follow the diet. My first question was an obvious one. Wouldn't anyone lose weight eating only 500 calories a day? The answer was equally obvious. Yes, anyone would lose weight eating only 500 calories a day, but considering that this number is only 25 to 30 percent of the average person's daily caloric intake, how long would a dieter be able to stick to this routine? I felt the hunger would simply be too much to bear.

It may sound silly, but my biggest source of resistance was probably the diet's prohibition of salad dressing. Would I really eat handfuls of salad greens with no dressing? Yuck. Could I actually survive for months on just a few types of greens that I didn't really like? I liked food too much to do that. Granted, this is, in part, the reason why I got fat, but I still felt a need to get some satisfaction from my food.

INVENTING MY OWN WHEEL

Drawing on my many years of writing about the subject of natural health and wellness, as well as numerous conversations with several knowledgeable friends and colleagues, including Frankie and Dr. Cass, I realized something that was little discussed in Dr. Simeons' time: The HCG diet is not only a precisely formulated low-calorie diet, it is also a low-fat, low-carbohydrate and low-glycemic-index eating plan. (See the inset "What Is the Glycemic Index?" on page 15.) If you stay within its parameters and get a little help from HCG, you will surely succeed. Your body will have no other choice but to burn its fat reserves in order to function. I was supremely confident that I would lose weight if I stuck to this plan, but my visceral reaction to the 500-calorie limit prompted me to choose a slightly different route to weight loss.

What Is the Glycemic Index?

The glycemic index is a system of measurement that ranks each food according to its effect on blood sugar levels. Foods such as broccoli and onions have very little effect on blood sugar levels and, therefore, also have very low glycemic index numbers. Conversely, pumpkins and parsnips each have high glycemic index numbers, as they raise blood sugar considerably. The information provided by this scale is invaluable to those who wish to lose weight, manage their diabetes, or reduce their risk of a number of other negative health conditions.

Instead of the 500-calorie-per-day method, I decided to eat 700 calories per day. I had found a number of sources that recommended this calorie level for long-term HCG dieters, of which I knew I would be one. I felt that this level was much more realistic, and that the extra 200 calories would likely have little effect on my weight loss. Unfortunately, I also knew that the additional 200 calories shouldn't include cheese—not even low-fat cheese—so I grimly bit the bullet and scratched cheese, a personal addiction, off my list.

Knowing I would be on the plan for the long haul, I began to prepare for my debut on the simplified HCG diet. I sculpted my own personalized version that would work for me. I found some helpful food charts to learn the calorie counts, fat amounts, carbohydrate values and glycemic index numbers of a wide variety of foods. (See the Calorie Counts on page 87 and the Glycemic Index Chart on page 91.) In light of the food restrictions, supplement prohibitions and beauty product exclusions associated with the Simeons Protocols, I knew I had a few issues to tackle in my own way if I truly wished to stick to the HCG diet. The following are the main items I addressed in my attempt to ease the process.

CARBOHYDRATES

When it comes to carbs, Dr. Simeons wants you to eat only those dry, nasty breadsticks made from white flour. I'm not sure why. I can only guess that, practicing in Italy more than sixty years ago, it would have been very difficult to put on the brakes in the face of all that soft, crusty Italian bread and delicious pasta. Perhaps breadsticks were the best alternative at the time. Today, however, there are some healthful and tasty whole grain breads and crackers on the market, including flatbreads and 100-calorie sandwich rounds. I even bought fairly heavy breads, slicing them thinly so that one piece was less than 100 calories. My main concern was always to keep my bread consumption to no more than 100 calories a day.

After starting the diet, I also found an occasional afternoon bowl of plain popcorn (only 100 calories for nearly five cups of popped kernels!) to be a welcome variation. Of course, that bowl fulfills the total carb allowance for the day, which is something to keep in mind. I also feel that 100 calories of any other carbohydrate, such as brown rice, would probably have been acceptable as well. Exercise your options whenever you feel the need. The most important point is to eat a whole grain carbohydrate for maximum nutrition and minimum effect on blood sugar levels.

COFFEE

Sure, Dr. Simeons says that you can drink all the black coffee you want while on the HCG diet. But what is coffee without half-and-half? I simply wasn't willing to give up drinking my coffee the way I wanted it. Trying to get around the problem, I discovered that, later in his practice, Dr. Simeons agreed that his patients could have one tablespoon of milk a day. In the interest of being able to sustain myself on a diet that I knew would last six months or more, I decided to make another trade-off. I adjusted the meal plan to allow two tablespoons (twenty calories) of fat-free half-and-half per day. As a sweetener, I decided to use stevia, which is a natural calorie-free sweetener derived from the stevia plant, instead of an artificial product such as Splenda.

The small adjustment to the half-and-half allowance improved my psychological well-being immensely. I truly believe that psychological well-being is critical to the success of this diet, so the change was more important than you may realize. Although, I admit, sometimes the line between psychological well-being and self-indulgence is hard to discern. OK, I'll plead guilty. My fat-free half-and-half was an indulgence. But it was one that had a positive effect on my attitude and almost no effect on my waistline, so I think it was more than worth it.

MEAT

I don't eat fish, so to avoid complete boredom with the steady cycle of beef and chicken, I occasionally added lean pork loin, egg, or tofu to the diet. As far as meat goes, lean meat is lean meat. There is little caloric or fat difference between a piece of sirloin steak, a piece of pork loin and a piece of chicken or turkey breast, provided they are carefully weighed while raw. I became pretty good at estimating portion sizes, actually. (A portion of meat is approximately the size of my hand, which is small.) It's a little game I played with myself. Nevertheless, I still weighed my meat on a scale to be absolutely sure. I even traveled with a small battery-operated scale.

SALAD DRESSING

I knew I wanted to allow myself a bit of salad dressing for my greens, but a cruise through the supermarket aisle showed me that most dressings are horrifically high in calories and fat. Thankfully, I discovered two brands that are low in calories and fat but still tasty. Walden Farms Sugar-Free Italian and several varieties from the Maple Grove Farms line of dressings (including balsamic vinaigrette, Caesar and

Greek) fit the bill. They are made entirely of healthful ingredients and have only ten calories for every two tablespoons. That's a miniscule trade-off for improved flavor and an enjoyable salad.

SKIN CREAMS

Don't get me started on skin creams! I would never give up my moisturizer. After all, I am a woman of a certain age and vain enough to want to stay as wrinkle-free as possible. I use good-quality organic skin care products and do not in any way scrimp on them while on the HCG diet, all without any apparent ill effects. I can only surmise that Dr. Simeons didn't know much about them, having so little information to work with in 1954.

A note about skin and wrinkling: Fat loss will most likely result in loose skin. To combat this problem, I dry brush my entire body after every shower. It stimulates circulation and lymphatic drainage. Be sure to brush in the direction of your heart, about eight strokes in each location, with special attention to your thighs, buttocks, belly and the backs of your arms. I also brush upwards on my neck, towards my face. You can use a natural bristle brush available at most bath shops or even in the cosmetics section of discount stores. Your brush should feel stimulating, but it shouldn't hurt you when used vigorously. I find that a brush with a handle is easiest to use.

Finally, although Dr. Simeons advises against massages, I have no idea why he does so, and I can't imagine how they could be harmful. I don't see a problem in deviating from that rule. Feel free to see if massages work for you. For many people, massages provide stress reduction, improved circulation and an overall feeling of well-being. Personally, I love massages for their self-nurturing effect.

SOUP

I don't care that much about soup in general, but remember that I started the HCG diet in November. It is cold in the mountains of

Western North Carolina where I live, and I think the low-fat nature of the diet made me feel cold all the time. My problem wasn't hunger pains, it was cold. I needed hot food! I made the decision to allow chicken and beef broth in my diet, so I started making soup. I found an excellent soup base called Better Than Bouillon, which is somewhat lower in sodium than most bouillon cubes but still has a rich, satisfying flavor—all that and just ten calories a cup. When I prepare soup, I generally add finely chopped cabbage, celery, onions, garlic, Portobello mushrooms and whatever other vegetable is around (often spinach, green beans, broccoli, kale, or cauliflower) to my broth.

I never use a recipe to make soup. I just eyeball everything and go with my gut. I usually sprinkle chopped cilantro or some other herb on top. My effort makes a full meal, with a big bowl coming in at about fifty to seventy calories per serving on average. Best of all, it is hot! Improvised meals such as this one are a compromise that did not hinder my fat-shedding plan one bit. They simply made it more likely that I would stay the course.

SPICES AND HERBS

What would food be without spices and herbs? Virtually all spices and herbs are either very low in calories or have no calories at all, so I always use them to my heart's content. I've recently been buying lettuce mixed with herbs that has loads of dill in it. It is delicious! The cilantro and parsley in my soup or salad, the rosemary or turmeric on my chicken and the cinnamon sprinkled on my baked apple made all the difference in keeping me interested, satisfied and able to carry on while on the diet. One thing I will point out, however, is this: When you buy a mix of any sort, you should always look at what's in it. Too much sodium or sugar—which comes under many different names, including fructose, sucrose and maltodextrin—can easily derail your diet. Ultimately, if you'd like to make your life easier, just avoid mixes altogether and create your own combinations from fresh or dried spices and herbs.

SUPPLEMENTS

The Simeons HCG diet prohibits the use of dietary supplements. I, however, agree with my friend Dr. Cass, who allows them. I suppose cutting out your daily supplements wouldn't matter much if you were only going to be on the diet for a month or so. But what if you continue the plan for six months or more?

Although the HCG diet is exceptionally healthy, it still has its nutritional shortcomings. For example, even if you are a fish eater, which I am not, you will not get sufficient omega-3 fatty acids from the white fish allowed in this program. I took fish oil capsules for my omega-3s while on the diet, and they didn't seem to cause any problems. Actually, I believe they helped my skin from becoming overly dry from the lack of fat in my meal plan.

In addition to omega-3s, I think everyone needs a good multivitamin. The American Medical Association (AMA) agrees with me on this subject. In addition, I find that a separate daily dose of B vitamins, particularly B_7 and B_{12}, provides important benefits. I also recommend taking magnesium, potassium and potassium iodide (iodine) supplements, and am a stout defender of daily curcumin capsules, which combat inflammation, the root of so many diseases. Finally, I endorse taking extra vitamin D_3, especially during the winter. The following is a list of supplements you absolutely should take not only while you're on the HCG diet but all the time.

■ **B Vitamins.** B vitamins help keep your energy up, which is a welcome aid when you're on the HCG diet. I take a B-complex vitamin, which includes all eight B vitamins in their appropriate ratios, as well as an additional 400 mcg of a sublingual form of B_{12}, which dissolves under the tongue. Some people like to get injections of B_{12} for a little extra energy, but I never felt a need to do that. About six months in to the diet, I added an extra 500 mcg of B_7, also called *biotin*, to my routine after I noticed some hair loss (the only side effect I experienced while on the diet), as it is known to encourage hair growth. B vitamins also promote a healthy immune system, improve nerve conductivity and help your brain produce the chemicals that prevent depression. These vitamins provide nutritional support for your eyes, hair, liver, brain, mouth, intestines, nerves, muscles and skin.

■ **Curcumin.** Curcumin, the active component in the spice turmeric, is thought to provide protection against disease, particularly cancer. The amazing thing about it is that it seems to inhibit the growth of cancerous cells while completely ignoring healthy cells. I think it is too important a supplement to abandon while on the diet. I recommend taking 400 mg of curcumin extract per day. Be sure to buy your curcumin extract in its highly absorbable form, BCM-95, in order to benefit fully from the supplement.

■ **Fish Oil.** Fish oil contains the omega-3 fatty acids known as *docosahexaenoic acid* (DHA) and *eicosapentaenoic acid* (EPA). In addition to offering other health benefits, these substances reduce inflammation in your body and have been associated with lowering blood pressure and heart rate. I take fish oil in capsule form. I recommend capsules that have an enteric coating, which allows them to dissolve only once they've reached the small intestine. This quality ensures proper absorption and eliminates the fishy belches that so often occur with these supplements. I suggest taking 1,000 mg of fish oil per day. If you're really hardcore about counting calories, two fish oil capsules represent about twenty calories. These extra calories might slow the progress of your diet by a day or two over a period of several months, but I wouldn't worry about such a minor amount. Finally, choose a brand of fish oil that has been purified so that you don't ingest any of the heavy metals common in fish these days.

■ **Magnesium, Potassium, Potassium Iodide (Iodine).** These minerals are all absolutely vital to cellular function, heart health and the proper activity of endocrine glands such as the thyroid. As a result, you should take them in supplement form while following such a restrictive diet. Aim to get approximately 420 mg of magnesium, 150 mcg of iodine and 4.7 grams of potassium every day.

■ **Multivitamins.** If you want to cover all your bases, I suggest taking a multivitamin. If possible, get one made from organic whole foods, which should ensure that your body absorbs the nutrients properly. In other words, I don't recommend getting a cheap multivitamin that costs ten dollars for a month's supply. While cost isn't an absolute gauge of quality, a product that is made from whole foods is generally a little more expensive than a synthetic brand, but the price is worth it. The nutrients in whole food brands tend to provide a synergistic effect that others do not.

The label on a bottle of multivitamins will show you the daily recommended value of each vitamin and mineral as recommended by the government, as well as the actual amount of each substance contained in the supplement. A high-quality vitamin will usually offer a handful of vitamins at a higher percentage than their daily recommended values (especially vitamins C and D and the B-complex vitamins) under the assumption that increased dosages of certain nutrients promote a healthy body. (Regardless of these higher values, however, I still take an extra B-complex vitamin in addition to my mutli for an extra boost of energy.) When it comes to supplements and their dosages, talk to your doctor if you have any concerns or questions before starting a multivitamin regimen. And feel free to add any other supplements your healthcare professional may suggest.

■ **Vitamin D.** Chicago physician and bestselling author Dr. Mayer Eisenstein is a big proponent of vitamin D as a weight-reduction aid. I agree with him and add that it helps with a myriad of health problems, including diabetes, several types of cancer, as well as hypertension and other forms of cardiovascular disease. As most of us are deficient in this vitamin, I recommend taking a daily supplement, especially during the winter, when the there is not enough sun to promote the natural production of vitamin D via UV exposure. I take 2,000 IU of vitamin D_3 daily, which is the most absorbable form of supplemental vitamin D available. Dr. Eisenstein actually suggests taking up to 10,000 IU a day, but you should have your blood levels of vitamin D checked first in order to determine how much you personally require.

VEGETABLES

I can't for the life of me understand why the Simeons Protocols so severely limit the types of vegetables allowed in the HCG diet, or why they allow only one type of vegetable to be eaten at any given meal. In addition to the spinach, chard, chicory, beet greens, salad greens, tomatoes, celery, fennel, onions, red radishes, cucumbers, asparagus and cabbage permitted by Dr. Simeons, I happily added green beans, broccoli, peppers, mushrooms and cauliflower to my diet. While I often ate my veggies raw, I also enjoyed steaming, roasting or braising them in a dry skillet with a little bit of broth to prevent moisture loss. As an occasional treat, I even ate spaghetti squash. In my opinion, any low-calorie, low-glycemic-index vegetable is fair game in just about any reasonable quantity. This, of course, rules out troublemakers such as potatoes, sweet potatoes, corn, carrots, peas and avocados. (Sorry!)

While the Simeons Protocols don't clearly specify a permissible amount of daily vegetables, I found approximately four cups of vegetables per day to be ideal. I usually divided that amount between lunch and dinner, so get your measuring cup out.

TAKING BREAKS AND BUILDING IMMUNITY

As for the recommended breaks associated with the Simeons HCG diet (a six-week hiatus from the diet before starting the program again), they are not necessary in the simplified version I've created. If you need to be on the diet for six months or more, you can continue on the plan until you reach your goal weight, provided you don't experience any serious side effects. Even if you decide to take time off from the diet, as I did over the holidays, you may simply continue to take HCG while avoiding sugar and carbohydrates as much possible, and keeping your calorie count low.

According to his version of the HCG diet, Dr. Simeons attributes the need for breaks to the theory that some people may build immunity to HCG over time. Although it doesn't seem to happen to everyone, one friend of mine who experienced this phenomenon while on the HCG diet said that the major symptom of her HCG desensitization was extreme hunger. She said it was so severe that she could have eaten her own pillow at night. I did not notice any personal immunity to HCG while on the diet, but was prepared to go on hiatus from the plan if such a thing developed, of course. I guess I would have recognized it as soon as my pillow started to look particularly tasty!

THE NAYSAYERS

There will be those who will say that a 700-calorie-per-day limit is too radical to be healthful. Your doctor will likely agree with that assertion if you are unfortunate enough to see a practitioner who knows little about nutrition and has knee-jerk reactions to new ideas. "You can't sustain life on so few calories. You will begin the starvation process and your muscles will waste away," people will tell you, conveying concern for your well-being. "Besides, no one ever keeps the weight off after one of these crash diets," they will add. If you get that attitude from your medical professional or even from your friends, just point to Dr. Simeon's book *Pounds and Inches*, which offers scientific research to back up the claims of the HCG diet. The book can also be downloaded online for free, so there is no reason the naysayers cannot discover the truth for themselves. (See the Resources on page 93.).

Next, ask the critics of this program if gastric bypass or lap band surgery is healthier than the HCG diet. Sure, medical professionals often recommend these types of procedures for the morbidly obese, but that doesn't mean they are better. In fact, people who have had gastric bypass or lap band surgery generally cannot take in more than 700 calories a day anyway. And for most of them, this fact remains true for the rest of their lives, whether they like it or not. How can it possibly be healthier for people to undergo surgery, with all its attendant drugs, risks associated with anesthesia and infection, as well as other complications? Surgery doesn't even provide the beneficial metabolic reset that HCG does. People who go through these procedures must be unbearably hungry, not to mention subject to daunting health consequences. Granted, I understand that the people who get these surgeries are desperate. I just wish they would all try HCG before going under the knife.

The truth is that, after more than sixty years of use, the HCG diet has been validated as a means of permanent weight loss. While the reasons behind HCG's effectiveness are not yet fully understood, it is thought that the hormone signals your body to burn fat but not muscle tissue, and then resets your metabolic rate to keep you at your goal weight. Whatever the exact scientific mechanism behind their weight loss, people on the HCG diet have a high success rate and a low incidence of putting the weight back on, assuming they follow the plan through the important final phase. There is no evidence of muscle wasting or any serious side effects that would be expected on a starvation diet. In fact, throughout the diet, your body learns to survive on the appropriate calorie count for your desired weight. It consumes fat—about 1,000 calories worth each day on average—to make up the deficit from the 700-calorie-per-day routine.

Most naysayers are just uninformed individuals reacting to something they do not understand. Since a large number of doctors have at best a few hours of nutrition education over the course of their medical training—and even less background in weight control and the mechanisms that affect it—it's not surprising that their only advice to overweight patients is to eat less and exercise more, or to opt for surgery.

Conclusion

If you don't think you have the willpower to follow the HCG diet, think again. HCG will be your willpower. HCG curbs your appetite, and the adjusted guidelines make the program so easy to manage that you will be able to stay on it for as long as it takes to reach your goal weight.

The truth is that most people *need* a program to help them drop extra weight and keep it off. While critics will just tell you to eat less and exercise more, that idea is too imprecise to be of any real help to most overweight people. If it were that simple, no one would have a weight problem. You need to know that there is a diet you can follow that is proven and sustainable, especially when the medical community is so quick to recommend weight-reduction surgery, which is rife with dangers. The simplified version of the HCG diet that I outline in this book is a safe and healthful alternative to gastric bypass and lap band procedures for those who need to shed a considerable amount of weight. I know because it worked for me.

3

What You Can Eat and What You Can't

I want to be sure you don't get the wrong idea. The Super Simple HCG Diet is still a stringent program with very specific "Do's" and "Don'ts." It's serious. You cannot take HCG, eat whatever you'd like and expect results. There is no such thing as a free lunch, as they say. The magic pill may be HCG, but it goes hand in hand with a deep commitment and real effort on your part. You must stick to the 700-calorie-per-day regimen to achieve a reduction in weight. (A tiny indulgence here and there, however, doesn't seem to be harmful, so try not to feel too intimidated).

You must also eat all of the mandatory foods on the diet every day. No, you can't swap out a ninety-calorie pear for an extra ninety-calorie piece of bread. (I found that out the hard way.) The HCG diet is about much more than just calories. While not all the scientific reasons behind the diet's effectiveness are understood, there seems to be a specific balance of meat, vegetables, fruit and carbohydrates that must exist for the HCG program to work. This chapter outlines the details of the diet, listing the prohibitions, allowances and strategies that helped me stay on target and lose weight.

WHY 700 CALORIES?

I think you'd probably do fine on the 500-calorie-per-day HCG diet if you had no more than twenty to twenty-five pounds to shed and were planning on following the program for only a month or so. In my opinion, however, eating 500 calories a day is too extreme to follow over the long-term, which, in my mind, is any period longer than thirty days. People on 500-calorie diets complain of low energy and describe themselves as weak, tired and fuzzy-brained. That's because 500 calories are simply not enough to sustain the human body over an extended period of time, with or without HCG. Bumping that number up to 700 calories is probably my diet's biggest deviation from the Simeons Protocols, and one that is endorsed by dozens of experts. I am so glad I decided to make the change.

It was an entirely different world at 700 calories. I slept less than I had before starting the diet. I worked with more focus. My energy level was noticeably higher. (I know all this because I sometimes found myself folding laundry and checking email at close to midnight.) I engaged in moderate exercise without any noticeable fatigue and my stamina seemed to consistently improve as I shed the pounds that had literally weighed me down for two decades.

According to reports I have read of other dieters who have made the same adjustment to the HCG plan, there seems to be no significant difference in weight loss between dieters on a 700-calorie-per-day regimen and dieters on a 500-calorie-per-day routine. I suspect that this is because a higher calorie level supports a higher activity level, and a higher activity level supports increased calorie burning.

THE FIRST TWO DAYS

As you learned in Chapter 2, fatty foods are highly recommended during the first two days of the HCG diet. I'll bet that you were pleased to discover this fact. From my lofty position as a successful longtime HCG dieter, this idea sounds strange and gross to me now, but it does appear necessary. The body's fat-burning mechanism seems to be triggered by a big forty-eight-hour fat binge. This means you get to eat French fries, burgers, ice cream, pizza, donuts and any other rich foods you'd like for two whole days. Get it into your system so you can get it out of your system, so to speak. You may, of course, choose not to follow this advice, particularly if you suffer from heart disease of high cholesterol, but the fat binge really does jumpstart the fat burn. It is the reason I was able to shed an amazing nine pounds in the first week of my HCG diet experience. Weight loss does not continue at this rapid rate, but the large initial drop in pounds is a fantastic psychological boost. By the third day of the diet, however, the restriction begins.

MEASURING YOUR FOOD

Measuring your food is the key to the HCG diet. Unfortunately, before starting the diet, I had a rather distorted view of what constitutes an appropriate portion size. In regard to the humongous plates of food dished out at almost every restaurant in the country, I think this incorrect perception is pretty common. Since most of us never really pay attention to the size of our meals, portion control is a skill that must be learned simply by doing it on a regular basis. Make it a habit until you get the hang of it.

Buy a food scale. Mine cost about fifteen dollars and is especially convenient because it allows me to weigh food directly on its clear glass plate. If you do not get one with a clear glass plate, make sure you get a scale that can be zeroed out with your own serving dish on it. This way you can place your food on the dish and place the dish on the scale without worrying about doing the math to determine exactly how much your food weighs *without* the dish. And as you already know, you should first remove all visible fat from any meat you weigh and, of course, weigh it raw. Don't leave anything to guesswork. Know exactly what is going into your body and you'll reap the results you desire. Even if you are mathematically challenged, the more you do it, the easier it will become.

The same goes for keeping a measuring spoon and a measuring cup handy. These tools are invaluable. They prevented me from overdoing the fat-free half-and-half as well as the salad dressing, and from underestimating my vegetable and fruit portions. Finally, use the Diet Diary on page 97 to log your daily food intake at each meal according to type of food, portion size and calorie count. You may also use it to record your hunger levels and any feelings you have. Keeping track of your experience can help you adjust to the HCG diet confidently. Success is truly a matter of basic arithmetic and personal reflection.

GLYCEMIC INDEX AND GLYCEMIC LOAD

As you know, the glycemic index measures the effect a food has on blood sugar levels. Foods that break down and release their natural sugars quickly into the bloodstream, like potatoes and corn, are high glycemic index foods. They are, therefore, not recommended. Low glycemic index foods, however, such as asparagus and broccoli, which have a milder effect on blood sugar, are all fair game in my version of the HCG diet. Simply consult a good glycemic index chart and eat only those items whose glycemic index number falls below fifty. (See the Glycemic Index Chart on page 91.)

If you'd like to be more exacting in your research, look up the glycemic load of your foods. (See the Resources on page 93.) The glycemic load is a measurement that takes into account both the speed with which the sugars in a food are released during digestion as well as the actual quantity of sugars contained in a serving of that food. While foods with low glycemic index numbers almost always have low glycemic loads, there are exceptions. Watermelon, for example, contains sugars that spike blood sugar levels rapidly.

Because watermelon is mostly water, however, the quantity of these sugars is very low. Thus, it has a high glycemic index number of about seventy but a low glycemic load of about four, which makes it an allowable food. If you limit your intake to foods with a glycemic load of ten or less, you will be fine.

THE "MUST EAT" LIST

The simplified version of the HCG diet offers considerably more latitude than Dr. Simeons' original routine—adding 200 calories to your daily intake and expanding the range of allowable foods—but still has certain rules that must be followed diligently, including a list of "must eat" foods. The following types of food are required, without fail, every day.

- ❑ Approximately four cups of vegetables from the "must eat" veggie list (See page 32)

- ❑ Two servings of fruit from the "must eat" fruit list (See page 33)

- ❑ Seven ounces of lean meat from the "must eat" meat list (See page 33)

- ❑ One 100-calorie portion of bread from the "must eat" bread list (See page 34)

- ❑ Sixty-four ounces of water (minimum)

Note that the only processed item included on the list is bread. I would strongly suggest that you opt for whole grain bread. Be a careful label reader and don't slip on this one! All of the required foods can be found in your local market. I also recommend that you buy organic meat, fish, fruits and vegetables whenever possible, if your pocketbook permits. The fewer chemicals you ingest from your food, the better off you will be.

As you may have noticed, each category of food has its own "must eat" list from which to create your meals. Although these food requirements limit your choices considerably, keep in mind that you can apportion your vegetables, fruit, meat, bread and water in any way you'd like. For example, if you'd prefer to have three cups of vegetables at dinner and only one at lunch, so be it. As long as you stick to the daily servings previously mentioned, the diet will work. True, there's not a whole lot of room for deviation, but there are a number of foods that you can eat in unlimited quantity, as you will see on page 34.

THE "MUST EAT" VEGGIE LIST

The vegetables below are not the only ones allowed, but they *are* the ones from which to choose when preparing your four cups of "must eat" veggies for the day. They may be bought fresh or frozen, but never canned or processed in any way.

- ❏ alfalfa sprouts
- ❏ asparagus
- ❏ artichokes
- ❏ beet greens
- ❏ bell peppers (all colors)
- ❏ broccoli
- ❏ Brussels sprouts
- ❏ cauliflower
- ❏ cabbage
- ❏ collard greens

- ❏ green beans
- ❏ kale
- ❏ mushrooms
- ❏ mustard greens
- ❏ red radishes
- ❏ spinach
- ❏ squash
- ❏ Swiss chard
- ❏ tomatoes

THE "MUST EAT" FRUIT LIST

As is the case with the vegetables, the fruits on the list below may be bought fresh or frozen. Consult a calorie chart for exact portion sizes, but generally one serving equals one medium-sized piece of fruit, or half a cup of berries or melon. The choices include:

- apples
- blackberries
- blueberries
- cantaloupe
- cherries
- clementines
- grapefruit
- grapes
- honeydew melon
- Mandarin oranges
- nectarines
- peaches
- pears
- raspberries
- strawberries
- watermelon

THE "MUST EAT" MEAT LIST

As you know, all meats must be extremely lean with all visible fat removed while still raw. Chicken and turkey should be boneless and skinless. Despite the restrictions, there are actually quite a variety of meats from which to choose, including:

- beef
- flank
- ground round (use 93-percent lean ground round if you'd like a burger occasionally)
- sirloin
- tenderloin
- top round
- tri-tip
- chicken breast

❑ fish

● cod

● crab

● flounder

● haddock

● halibut

● lobster

● sea bass

● tilapia

● shrimp

❑ pork loin

❑ turkey breast

THE "MUST EAT" BREAD LIST

While you might wish to swap out your bread allowance for some rice or pasta, I did not do so while on the diet, according to advice I'd received. I had no evidence to prove that the substitution would disrupt the success of the diet, but I chose to designate the list below as my "must eat" options. Whatever your decision, always check the calorie count of everything you buy. I personally got my daily 100 calories of bread products from:

❑ multigrain sandwich rounds

❑ multigrain tortillas

❑ non-fat whole grain bread

❑ whole grain flat bread

UNLIMITED FOODS

If you're starting to think that the HCG diet is a little grim, dull and boring, don't despair. There are plenty of little ways to give a zing to your food and keep your taste buds interested. There are a number of foods that you can eat to your heart's content, including:

- [ ] all herbs and spices
- [ ] celery
- [ ] dill pickles
- [ ] garlic
- [ ] hot sauce
- [ ] jarred jalapeños and other hot peppers
- [ ] lemons
- [ ] limes
- [ ] mustard (be sure the label reads zero calories)
- [ ] onions
- [ ] salad greens
- [ ] tea
- [ ] vinegar
- [ ] Worcestershire sauce

I found celery quite a satisfying snack, probably because of its crunch. And celery actually has negative calories, meaning your body uses more calories to digest celery than the food provides, so feel free to eat as many stalks as you'd like.

If a little vinegar on your salad isn't good enough, you can try sugar-free non-fat salad dressing. As you know, the only brands I personally find suitable are Walden Farms and Maple Grove Farms of Vermont, which have five to ten calories per two-tablespoon serving. These dressings are a boon for big salads, which are a staple of my life. They can add a great deal of variety to what can become an extremely bland and boring diet. If you wish to try a different brand, simply check the calorie count of your choice of dressing to be sure it falls below ten calories per serving. Remember, you still have to measure!

INDULGENCES

As I mentioned in the last chapter, when I learned that the original HCG diet doesn't allow half-and-half to be added to coffee, I became concerned. I felt the point could possibly be a deal breaker. So, I decided to make a daily exception to the rule, allowing myself two tablespoons of fat-free half-and-half per day. It is little indulgences such as this one that can be invaluable to the success of the diet, I believe. They prevent you from feeling as though you're in a constant state of denial, which can be a recipe for failure.

Substituting plain popcorn for your bread portion is also a great way to feel a bit decadent every now and then. And although an indulgence such as alcohol isn't a necessity for me, it is nice to have a glass of wine on occasion if I'm out with friends. (Remaining sociable and connected to friends helps more than you know.) As long as you ensure that the serving size remains under 100 calories, the following items are indulgences that may be added to your daily diet every once in a while.

- ❏ Five cups of air-popped popcorn without butter (substitute for bread portion that day)

- ❏ Five ounces of dry wine (no sweet wines)

- ❏ One low-calorie beer

- ❏ One shot of distilled spirits (check calorie count to be sure that one shot does not exceed 100 calories. Of course, you must use a no-calorie mixer.)

- ❏ Two tablespoons of fat-free half-and-half

Aside from the above, no other indulgences are permitted on the simplified version of the HCG diet. Even these should be enjoyed on a very occasional basis. Other than the fat-free half-and-half, which I allow daily, I do not recommend including these indulgences more than twice a week. This suggestion goes for the alcoholic beverages in particular, as the extra 100 calories per day they contribute can slow your weight loss. And no, you can't eat fewer veggies and more popcorn, or consider wine a "fruit," as tempting as it might be to do so.

WHAT ABOUT SWEETENERS?

As you can see, the diet doesn't permit the use of table sugar, honey, maple syrup or any other high-calorie sweetener. But what about calorie-free artificial sweeteners? Well, from my years of being a health writer, I've learned a few things about these substances. I don't recommend aspartame (Equal) or saccharin (Sweet'N Low) in any amount. There is sufficient scientific evidence to confirm that these products are hazardous to your health and may even ruin your diet. As for sucralose (Splenda), the jury is still out. I personally like it, and researchers I trust have said it is all right as long as you keep your consumption modest. That being said, this sweetener also has its critics. Ultimately, the choice is yours.

While stevia has been available in the United States for two decades, it has only recently been allowed to be marketed as a no-calorie sweetener. Advertised as a natural sweetener under a number of names, including Truvia and Sweet Leaf, stevia may be a healthier alternative to the other sweeteners mentioned above. It comes from a natural plant source and, according to some scientific evidence, may actually help control blood sugar levels.

THE "MUST NOT EAT" LIST

Now that you know which foods you *must* eat and which foods you can eat, it's time to learn which foods you absolutely *cannot* eat while on the HCG diet. The following list details the foods I gave up for the sake of weight loss.

- ❑ baked goods
- ❑ bread (except the low-calorie whole grain versions mentioned on page 34)
- ❑ carrots
- ❑ cheese

- ❏ corn

- ❏ high-fructose corn syrup

- ❏ milk and milk products (except the fat-free amount allowed for your coffee or tea)

- ❏ pasta

- ❏ peas

- ❏ potatoes (including sweet potatoes and other root vegetables)

- ❏ processed foods (except for bread and salad dressing)

- ❏ sauces (except those made from the approved ingredients in their allowed quantities)

- ❏ sugar

- ❏ yogurt

As an appealing alternative to pasta, I often used spaghetti squash. Keep in mind that most salad dressings contain high-fructose corn syrup or sugar, which is not recommended. Try to seek out the brands I mentioned earlier, or pick one that stays below ten calories a serving. Finally, does all this information mean that pizza is on the forbidden list? Sadly, it does.

FOOD SHOPPING AND COOKING

As you know, you should lean toward organic foods as much as possible. You are already paying such close attention to the foods you're putting in your body, so why would you want unknown chemicals entering your system? While organic foods can be vastly more expensive, they are, in many cases, worth the expense. But, of course, look at your budget and make the decision based on what you are willing to do and what you *can* do. Although you're buying more expensive produce and cuts of meat, your grocery bill will likely be lower than it once was, simply because you are eating less. In addition, you may be able to grow much of your own food during the summer months, reducing your grocery bill even more. If you cannot grow your own, farmers' markets are great sources of nutritious produce.

In regard to cooking methods, you won't be frying anything. All of your meat will be grilled, broiled, baked, steamed or braised. Personally, on or off the diet, I braise my choice of meat in a ceramic-coated frying pan, adding a couple of tablespoons of chicken, beef or veggie stock when the meat does not retain enough moisture of its own. I often cook my veggies right in the same pan for a faux stir-fry.

Conclusion

Trust me, after a while you will find that the rules of this diet are logical and simple. Once this happens, you will feel a creative spark and want to try a few new variations, add a few spices, and perk up your taste buds. The simplicity of this version of the HCG diet is actually a large part of its beauty. I quickly learned to savor the flavors of each food as nature created it, minus all the sauces, sugar, butter and cheese. I now find that I truly enjoy these foods and, as a result, my hankering for unhealthful meals has faded tremendously. I truly believe that anyone can attain the same result from this lifestyle.

4

Shots or Drops?

The Simeons Protocols call for the use of HCG doses administered via syringe. Of course, the idea of daily injections frightens many people. I completely understand, because it certainly frightened me. The first time I had to poke myself with a needle, I was scared to death. But I got over it and so can you. If you are truly against using a needle, though, there is now an alternative that wasn't available in Dr. Simeons' time. In addition to describing the HCG options at your disposal, this chapter discusses where you might find a doctor who can help you with the program. It also lists the medical conditions that make the HCG diet inadvisable.

NEEDLES, SYRINGES AND SHOTS, OH MY!

Let's talk about injections first. If you feel flutters in your stomach every time you think of the subject, I can help you overcome them. If you choose to take HCG by injection, let me reassure you: As you do it on a daily basis, the shots will become a lot easier. The process is a little like wearing contact lenses for the first time. The first week of putting them in and taking them out is tough, but soon you're doing it without even thinking. The more you use the syringe, the less intimidating it is.

If you've never given yourself shots of any kind before, ask your doctor or a nurse to show you how it's done. You'll feel much more comfortable with the idea once the mystery has been removed. You'll be injecting 100 to 125 international units (IU) of HCG into your belly fat every day. (I tended to do it in the morning, simply because I found it easy to remember to take the shot at this time of day.) You'll be using a 1-cc (cubic centimeter) insulin syringe with a 30-gauge needle, which is a little thicker than a hair, measuring five-sixteenths of an inch in length. Before using the needle, swab your belly with a sterile alcohol wipe. I recommend using one that contains a tiny bit of the local anesthetic *lidocaine*. This should numb the area enough so that you don't even feel the little pin prick.

Prior to following the HCG diet, I was no stranger to the practice of administering injections. I'd given hundreds of shots to my cats, dogs, horses and even to other humans. Before the HCG diet, however, I'd never given one to myself. In light of this fact, on the day I started the diet, I came downstairs full of determination. My HCG was mixed (I used a powdered form that must be mixed with a sterile water called *bacteriostatic water* and then refrigerated) and ready to go. I was all set. I walked to the cupboard and got out the first syringe. That's when I lost my nerve and my brain went into overdrive. "Maybe I don't really want to do this diet; maybe the injections are dangerous; maybe I'll give myself an infection; maybe it is simply too hard," I thought.

Sadly, I've performed this kind of self-sabotage on many occasions throughout my life. Fortunately, on that fateful day, I recognized my self-destructive habit and mentally shouted to myself, "BS!" I've gone scuba diving in five-mile deep waters. I've jumped out of airplanes. I've embarked on a vision quest in the wilderness and had jackals around my camp. I've covered wars and witnessed important historical events. I couldn't give myself a tiny little shot? "BS!" I mentally shouted to myself, even louder this time. I sat down, dropped my jeans, swabbed my belly with alcohol, drew up 100 IU of HCG into the syringe, gritted my teeth and stuck the needle in. It was over in seconds. I barely felt it. What an anticlimax! What a drama queen I had been! So, I admit, there was a moment of panic. But I overcame it. Now my morning injection is a part of my routine, like washing my face, brushing my teeth or weighing myself.

I chose to take HCG via injection for no particular reason other than that was the method made available to me. This option, however, won't be available to you unless you see your doctor or visit a medical spa that has an in-house doctor, since the shots require a prescription and should be followed under a doctor's supervision. Even if you do get a prescription, a doctor-supervised course of injections can be fairly costly, ranging anywhere from eighty to two thousand dollars per month. If this option does not seem viable, there is another way to get your daily dose of HCG.

ORAL HCG DROPS

If you cannot or will not inject yourself with HCG, maybe oral HCG drops are the way to go. HCG drops contain a diluted amount of the hormone and are administered orally via a standard dropper. Although they don't technically adhere to the principles of homeopathic medicine, oral HCG drops are often called "homeopathic" because they are prepared using the same dilution method employed by such pharmaceuticals. Like HCG injections, HCG drops can have a profound effect on weight loss. Although I chose not to use oral HCG, I know it works because I have seen results in those close to me. My daughter dropped ten pounds in the first two weeks on the diet using HCG drops, as did my friend Margaret. Granted, I think both of them suffered from hunger slightly more than I did at the outset, but the cravings were quickly stopped by an increase in dosage for a few days (from thirty drops to about sixty drops daily, with extra doses taken whenever hunger returned). Should you opt for this method, I recommend that you put the HCG drops in a glass of water to sip throughout the day. This should help curb cravings by keeping the dosage at a steady level.

There are, of course, a variety of opinions out there about oral drops—too many, in fact, to describe in this book. Suffice it to say, I think many of the objections to this form of HCG stem from ignorance of its effectiveness. Simply put, the proof is in the pudding. I've seen oral HCG reduce or eliminate hunger, help weight loss in target areas—including the buttocks, belly and thighs—and result in substantial decreases in waistline measurements. In fact, drops have certain advantages over injections. Some of these products feature additional hunger-suppressing and energizing ingredients, including l-glutamine, an amino acid that cuts cravings. In addition, they eliminate the need to stick a needle in your stomach, which can be a major stumbling block for a great number of people. Finally, they are often cheaper (usually around fifty dollars or less for a month's supply) than injections and can easily be bought online without a prescription. But buyer, beware! There are, unfortunately, many fake products out there. I suggest you buy your drops from someone you know or a reputable source that has been recommended to you. (See the Resources on page 93.)

CONSULTING YOUR REGULAR PHYSICIAN

If you choose to take HCG orally, technically you don't need the supervision of a doctor, but I still think your physician should be involved, especially if you're planning to drop more than fifteen pounds. In addition, talk to your doctor before starting the diet if you have any chronic health problems, as certain conditions make the HCG diet inadvisable. These conditions include:

❏ any condition that requires antibiotics

❏ cancer not in remission

❏ cancer being treated with chemotherapy

❏ gallbladder colic

❏ hypertension (high blood pressure) that requires two or more drugs to control

❏ hypotension (low blood pressure)

❏ infections occurring during the diet

❏ pregnancy or breastfeeding

❏ tuberculosis

❏ unstable angina

❏ unstable gout

❏ unstable, or "brittle," diabetes

❏ untreated Graves Disease

❏ a weak or compromised immune system

If you are taking any prescription medications, consult a physician before following the HCG diet. As noted by my friend Dr. Cass, the rapid weight loss experienced on the diet may affect the dosages of pharmaceuticals such as thyroid, blood pressure and diabetes medications, as well as hormone replacements. Have your blood levels checked every few weeks to determine if your prescriptions need adjustment. You may be pleasantly surprised, in fact, to learn that the dosages of your medications should be reduced. But please don't discontinue or reduce any medications on your own, no matter how you may feel.

FINDING A DOCTOR TO SUPERVISE YOUR HCG PROGRAM

Your primary care doctor may be willing to supervise your weight management program. If your physician is not familiar with HCG, you can recommend this book for further information. You can also encourage your doctor to contact other medical practitioners who have supervised the HCG diet successfully. Oftentimes, however, you will have to seek out a physician who is already familiar with the diet.

So, how do you find a doctor to supervise the HCG program? I wish I could give you a simple answer to the question. Sadly, there is no simple answer. Plug your city, state and the term "HCG" into an online search engine and you will likely get more than a few hits. But how will you know if these doctors are any good? That's the big question. A better bet, in my opinion, would be to ask around. Talk to your friends and your friends' friends. Post queries on online message boards that deal with HCG dieting. In addition, there are many medical spas that offer the HCG diet. If you can find one that has a medical or naturopathic doctor, I think it would be worth booking a consultation to see if the physician inspires confidence and feels like a good fit. And don't be afraid to ask to talk to other patients who have gone through the program under the doctor's supervision.

Be aware that supervised HCG programs are usually expensive and, in most cases, your insurance will not pay for them unless you have a medical condition that urgently requires weight reduction. Even in that case, it is more likely that your insurance will pay for a gastric bypass or lap banding, which can cost at least ten times as much as the HCG plan. While the HCG diet is safe, effective and simple, and no serious or lasting side effects have ever been reported, it is always best to have a doctor's guidance as you progress. I think your body, your health and your future are worth the investment, though I recognize that supervised care will simply not be possible for some people. Happily, the oral HCG drops are fairly inexpensive and easy to acquire.

FOR WOMEN ONLY

Despite what you may think, the HCG diet is intended for both sexes. At the moment, though, I must add a little section here just for women that deals with the use of HCG during a menstrual period, since I've gotten a number of questions about it.

Dr. Simeons recommends that women stop taking HCG but remain on the low-calorie diet during menstrual periods. I believe this is antiquated information. Today, most women choose to continue injections or drops during their periods, and I agree with their decision. There are, however, a couple of important facts to acknowledge in regard to the diet's effectiveness during this time of the month. Specifically, you may not continue to shed fat. In fact, you might gain a pound or two, even if you remain faithful to the diet. Do not be concerned. The weight loss will resume after your period, and may even accelerate a bit.

If you have a period that is heavier than normal, consult your doctor. The dosage of HCG should not be enough to cause menstrual problems, but everyone is unique. This is a good reason to have medical supervision while you're on the diet, even if you're using drops.

Conclusion

Ultimately, whether you choose injections or oral drops, or whether you follow the diet under a doctor's supervision or on your own, you will succeed as long as you stick to the meal plan. The trick is to overcome any anxiety you might have about the diet. Once you get started, a routine will click into place, as it did for me, and what once seemed intimidating will appear simple. The first step was the hardest and most worrisome for me, as I imagine it will be for you. It is natural to feel this way. But please understand that fear of the unknown can disappear in the blink of an eye, or the poke of a needle.

5

When the Time Is Right

You, and *only* you, will know when the time is right to begin the HCG diet. Part of the decision depends upon feeling psychologically and physiologically ready. The other part depends upon your schedule. In order for your new eating program to become a well-established aspect of your daily routine, you must start the diet at a time when there will be minimal distractions, temptations and potential stumbling blocks. That being said, I also want to remind you that there will be no absolutely "perfect" moment to begin, so avoid the procrastination trap and set a date as soon as possible. This chapter details my experience setting a date for the diet, deciding what my target weight should be, and gathering the tools I would require to succeed. It also offers advice on how best to take these first steps towards a fitter and healthier body.

SETTING A DATE

Ultimately, I started the program when I believed it was time. It was as simple as that. I felt it in my bones and knew that I would succeed. After making the decision to follow the HCG diet, I set my start date about three months in the future, planning it around a family wedding and an upcoming vacation. But, as I've already said, no time will ever be perfect. In my case, a week after I started the diet, my husband had to undergo back surgery. It wasn't expected to be a big deal, but it turned into a major medical issue, with several trips to the emergency room and an epic day of nightmares that ended in a second surgery. Thankfully, through it all, I remained absolutely committed to my diet. I ate some yucky salad and some even yuckier non-fat dressing in the hospital cafeteria and soldiered on, despite several enormously stressful days. Yes, I lapsed a couple of times, but I still shed six pounds that second week. The thrill of success spurred me on.

When you are ready, I suggest that you go to your calendar, choose a day that will work for you, and put a big red circle around the date. Set your cell phone to remind you. Talk to your family and enlist their support. This will be your D-day. This will be the day you begin your journey. Of course, be mindful of major stressors that might challenge your focus, like a big deadline at work, and do your best to avoid placing your start date too close to these potential stumbling blocks. In addition, travel, eating out and socializing are exceedingly difficult to manage during the early weeks of the HCG diet, so try to begin the plan at a time when you do not foresee any mandatory celebrations to attend, at least for the first six weeks or so. Finally, women of child-bearing age are advised to start the diet on the first day of menstruation.

DECIDING ON A TARGET WEIGHT

Once you've chosen a date, the next step is to decide on a target weight. If you haven't yet looked at a Body Mass Index (BMI) chart, now is the time to do so. (See the BMI Chart on page 51.) BMI measures weight in relation to height, resulting in a number that falls within a category on the BMI table. The categories range from "Underweight" to "Obese" and should give you a pretty good idea of your present weight level, as well as a healthful weight for your height. The recommended BMI is between 18.5 and 25 on the scale. Although the BMI chart does not take into account every factor concerning your weight, such as the size of your frame, it can give you a general idea of your current status. If you can recall the last time you were at your target weight (maybe you were a teenager), you will probably remember yourself as a more energetic, healthy, active and confident person. You can go back there, and you will!

BMI CHART

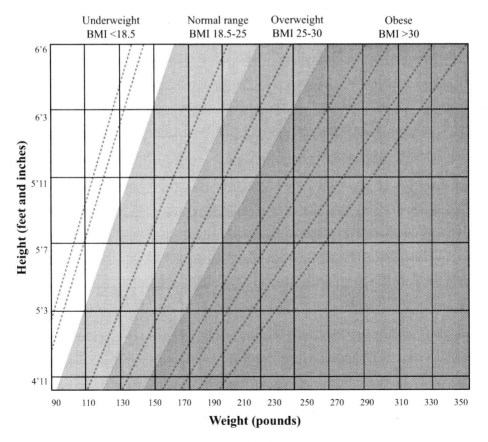

Once you know your goal weight, give yourself a rough estimate of how long it will take to shed the excess pounds. At the beginning, I estimated a required weight loss of twenty pounds per month for about six months, factoring in a couple of breaks (one for winter holidays and one for a time when I knew I would be traveling). I later revised this projection, slowing the weight loss as I went further along on the diet and had less to lose. Instead of twenty pounds per month, I aimed to get rid of twelve to fifteen pounds per month. I wasn't in a hurry, so I figure I had the freedom to let it take as long as it would take. It took me a little over eight months to drop 100 pounds. The feeling of euphoria I experienced upon reaching my goal was indescribable. I now possess the confidence to achieve and maintain an appropriate body size for the rest of my life.

GATHERING YOUR TOOLS

Once you've got your start date and target weight set, it is time to pick up a food scale, clean out your pantry (that doesn't mean you should eat everything in it!) and order your HCG. Next, go shopping for the necessary foods. (See Chapter 3.) I bought quite a bit of chicken and some steak, measured them out in three-and-a-half-ounce portions and froze them for convenience. Any advanced preparation that you are able to do will make your life that much easier while you're on the diet, which is a good thing.

If your family doctor has been receptive regarding your diet plan, or you have found a physician who specializes in the HCG diet, schedule a check-up. It will be interesting to see your cholesterol, triglyceride and blood pressure readings before your diet and compare them to the healthier levels that are sure to appear after the program. In addition, start a modest exercise routine or adjust the one you are already following. Thirty minutes of walking or gentle yoga every day will boost your energy without upsetting the balance of the fat-burning mechanism associated with HCG.

Finally, use the Diet Diary on page 97 to log your food intake according to food type, portion size and calorie count. You can also take note of your hunger levels, feelings, exercise habits and any stress management techniques used over the course of the diet. This information will serve as a helpful roadmap along the path to a slimmer, healthier you.

Conclusion

The most important thing you can do right now is start thinking about the program. Get yourself psychologically prepared. Visualize your success. I spent inordinate amounts of time perusing catalogs and websites for clothing and hairstyles that I would be able to wear once I reached my goal. I used many mental triggers, including picturing my closet void of all my fat clothes. In fact, now that I am 100 pounds lighter, nothing from my wardrobe fits. I am having great fun sweeping everything out of my closet, although there have been a few sentimental pieces that brought a little tear to my eye.

Positive visualization can benefit your cause immensely, but there is no substitute for an actual helping hand. In other words, look for a buddy. Believe me, moral support can be invaluable during the HCG diet. Never underestimate the power of friends. Finally, on your start date, wake up and congratulate yourself. You will have taken the first step on this journey, and it is by far the biggest and hardest one. Yes, there will be bumps in the road. There will likely be times when you falter, but your determination, careful planning and inner confidence will inspire you and help you stay on track. You will know when the time is right to begin, and this knowledge will make all the difference.

6

HCG Is for Men Too!

The idea of a man taking pregnancy hormone shots to lose weight seems ridiculous, right? Not really. As it turns out, men have achieved excellent results on the HCG diet. One of the most successful cases is California physician and author Dr. Mayer Eisenstein, who shed 100 pounds in just four months! The truth is that men are naturally leaner and lose weight more easily than women. It's not fair, my female friends, but it *is* a biological fact of life. Women have trouble losing weight because their bodies are simply better at storing fat. Through natural selection, our female ancestors developed this ability as a biological tool to deal with famine. Because fewer men are required to carry on the human race (I'm not in any way being anti-male here, so don't get riled up, guys!), it was women who evolved to carry the extra body fat needed to ensure their survival and, thus, the survival of the species. In other words, evolution gave women an advantage over men—at least it *was* an advantage at the time!

This theory explains Dr. Eisenstein's ability to drop 100 pounds in just four months. (He stuck pretty closely to the 500-calorie

Simeons Protocols, as far as I am aware.) In researching men and HCG, it seems that males are able to lose about one pound a day, which is approximately twice the rate expected in women over the long-term. I swear, I think my husband could get rid of five pounds just by skipping lunch! Despite knowing that the HCG diet can be even more effective for males, I have no doubt that men will require further reassurance before committing to the program.

COMMON QUESTIONS

As I just said, if you're a man, you probably have a list of questions you'd like answered regarding the HCG diet. In all honesty, I don't blame you. I know that if I were told that a male hormone could make me lose weight, I'd have questions, too. Having been asked a number of these queries by male friends, I would like to offer the following information to help ease your mind.

WILL MEN EXPERIENCE BIOLOGICAL FEMINIZATION?

"If HCG is a pregnancy hormone, won't I grow breasts or develop a high, squeaky voice?" This is the most common question posed to me by every one of my male friends. Guys, here's the answer to your burning question: No. In fact, some body builders use HCG not for weight loss but to kick start testosterone production, and in much greater amounts than recommended by the HCG diet. (Although, I don't suggest that you do the same.)

ISN'T HCG PRODUCED ONLY BY PREGNANT WOMEN?

While pregnant women certainly have elevated levels of HCG, the hormone is naturally produced by both men and non-pregnant women. In fact, HCG is a fertility hormone that is commonly prescribed to help women produce eggs and to strengthen sperm production in men. It is FDA approved to assist both sexes with conception and administered in much larger doses than those used in connection with the HCG diet. The HCG diet shouldn't affect your fertility, though, as the daily dosage of the hormone is so low. If you absolutely wish to avoid pregnancy while you're on the diet, you might want to take extra precautions to reduce the possibility of a surprise. If you're already pregnant or suspect that you may be pregnant, stop using HCG.

Is HCG Safe for Men?

According to the evidence, HCG is not only safe for men but also beneficial in many ways. You could say they thrive on it. Men lose weight at a lightning pace, decrease their cholesterol levels, lower their heart rates, and display reductions in blood pressure while on HCG treatments. These are huge advantages in terms of increasing overall health and longevity. Are there any major side effects from the hormone? No, there do not appear to be any serious side effects in men or women. Of course, HCG shots are associated with a slight risk of pain and soreness at the site of the injection, and even an abscess if you are not scrupulous about disinfection. Some men have complained about restlessness, but I suspect that the issue is due to an unfamiliar increase in energy brought about by the regimen rather than a true side effect.

ONE MAN'S STORY

My friend Jim very proudly lost fifty-six pounds in just forty-five days using the HCG diet. (Ladies, don't weep!) Here's how he did it: He received a bottle of drops that had been recommended by his doctor and, as Jim says, "kind of shoved it aside and forgot about it for a few weeks." Not long after, while watching television, he saw a story on the local news about a clinic that was charging $12,000 for a series of HCG treatments. (That's about ninety dollars a day!) The story got Jim's attention. He knew he had the bottle of drops sitting in his medicine cabinet and thought, "Why not give it a try?"

The first three or four days were "pretty tough," according to Jim. "I was drinking chicken bouillon four or five times a day, but after those first few days, I settled in to a fairly straightforward routine." He shed ten pounds in the first week. In his estimation, the amount of weight lost "was a phenomenal reward that made it easier to stay on the diet." He stayed on the diet for forty-five days, until the bottle ran out. During that time, his weight fell from 285 pounds to 229 pounds. His waist went from forty-five inches to forty inches. Jim admits to regaining eighteen pounds since going off the diet, but blames those few pounds on the fact that he did not follow the diet long enough to reset his default base weight, which, as you know, happens only after the completion of phase three.

Jim plans to start the diet again and drop another thirty to forty pounds when the time is right. It is only a matter of time before he blazes past me in number of pounds lost.

TIPS FOR SUCCESS

Based on his experience with the HCG diet, Jim has kindly offered me a few tips to pass on to both my male and female readers who may be curious about the program.

■ **Choose a Time When You Can Focus.** Be sure to start the diet only when you can focus completely on food for a few days. This is because the diet requires an all-consuming effort until you settle in to a routine. As I suggested in the last chapter, don't begin the program at a time when you foresee pressing work deadlines, holiday gatherings or other stressors ahead.

■ **Don't Sweat It.** Don't sweat the mistakes. We all make mistakes, and Jim himself admits to grabbing a cookie when his wife was baking, or eating a double portion of meat at dinner. Yes, cheating will slow or even stop your weight reduction, but it is not the end of the world. Start over.

■ **Weigh Yourself Daily.** Weighing yourself daily can keep you from cheating by reminding you that such indiscretions end up reflected on the bathroom scale. It also provides immediate gratification when you shed weight. Jim marks his weight on a calendar every day. I initially weighed myself on a weekly basis, thinking that a big weekly reading would be a more powerful psychological boost than an incremental daily reduction. After buying a fancy new digital scale, which measures weight loss to the nearest tenth of a pound, I too began to weigh myself daily!

■ **Try Those Tight Pants On.** This is a great tip for everyone. Buy a pair of pants that is too small for you and keep them in your closet. Once a week, try them on. You'll be pleasantly surprised at how little time it takes for the pants to fit you. (And soon they'll be too loose!) You may not notice a major change in the number on your scale each morning, but you will almost always feel a difference in the way the pants fit, which lets you know that you are still trimming inches off your waistline.

Conclusion

Yes, there are pitfalls associated with every diet, whether you are male or female. While men and women each experience some unique challenges, actively seeking support from other dieters, being aware of what lies ahead and planning for foreseeable stumbling blocks will help ensure your success. The next chapter tells you what form these challenges are likely to take and reveals ways to deal with each one.

7

Navigating the Potholes

I f you are lucky enough to have only twenty or twenty-five pounds to lose, you'll probably find the HCG diet experience to be very short and sweet. You could be done with the HCG shots or drops in four to six weeks, finish resetting your default weight in another three weeks and then get on with your life. Whatever length of time you choose to stay on the diet, I can confidently say that you are probably going to run into situations that will sidetrack you or even stop you in your tracks. These potholes are even more likely to appear if you're like me and have lots of weight to shed. In light of this fact, I'd like to offer a few thoughts to help you stay on track and continue marching towards your target weight.

FROM THE START

The first four to six weeks of the diet are a time of major physical and mental adjustment. The best advice I can give you is to be kind to yourself in the face of the challenges that arise. Before problems crop up, however, an awareness of what may lie ahead can make these issues less surprising and, as a result, a little easier to handle.

UNEXPECTED DETOX

Depending on your previous eating habits, your new healthful meal plan may trigger some symptoms of detoxification, usually within the first week of your diet. As your body begins to burn its fat reserves, it will also release the toxins that have built up in your tissues over the years. Once these substances are released, you may experience a number of symptoms, including headaches, fatigue and diarrhea. You may even think you have the flu. Don't let these symptoms dissuade you from the diet. They are a part of your body's natural process of eliminating the toxins contained in the unhealthful foods you were consuming. While the process is not pleasant, it is also not dangerous. It just means the diet is working. To help flush out the poison and speed up the detoxification process, be sure to drink plenty of water and rest whenever you feel the need.

HUNGER PANGS

Some people tell me that they feel hungry for the first couple of days of the diet. This is not a matter of concern, since the HCG may need time to build up in your system before it begins to curb your appetite. To alleviate these hunger pangs, drink more water and use the Emotional Freedom Technique. (See the inset "How to Stop Cravings Using the Emotional Freedom Technique" on page 64.) In addition, if you are using oral HCG drops, you can increase your dosage to sixty drops and add it to a glass of water to periodically sip throughout the day. This should keep your level of HCG consistent, possibly helping to prevent hunger. Do not increase your HCG dosage if you are taking injections of the hormone.

FEAR OF FAILURE

The human mind is an amazing thing. Thoughts like, "I can't do this," "It's too hard" or "Who am I trying to kid?" can wreak havoc on your willpower. This type of negative thinking can destroy your effort in so many ways, using fear to divert you from a path that will benefit you in the long-term. Don't be a victim of your own mind. To prevent a potential meltdown, I recommend meditation. Fifteen minutes a day will go a long way towards quieting a fearful mind.

There are literally hundreds of books on the subject, and almost as many forms of meditation from which to choose. I personally like the Buddhist technique and the meditative aspects of Kripalu yoga. (See the Resources on page 93.)

FEELING COLD

My biggest complaint during my time on the diet was that I almost always felt cold. Of course, I began the diet in winter, and, as you know, it is cold in the mountains where I live. But I do believe that my chilly body temperature was almost certainly due to the low-calorie nature of the diet and the fact that I ate almost no fat while on it.

Soup, hot tea and extra clothes were my answers to the problem. Sometimes I even wore my silk long johns. They fit perfectly under my increasingly baggy jeans. In hindsight, it might have been better to begin the diet in summer, when my garden provides wonderful organic produce. But that's just not how it happened. I have no regrets, though.

THE BREAKFAST CHALLENGE

The Super Simple HCG Diet doesn't lend itself very well to the traditional North American concept of breakfast. I know doctors will tell you that breakfast is the most important meal of the day, but unless you're into eating salads for breakfast or want to use your bread allowance first thing in the morning (which I didn't!), there really isn't much to eat for breakfast except a cup of coffee or tea, a piece of fruit or maybe a bowl of vegetable soup. These options

How to Stop Cravings Using the Emotional Freedom Technique

Developed by Gary Craig, the Emotional Freedom Technique (EFT) involves repeating an affirmation and tapping acupuncture points to desensitize a particular psychological or physical issue—in this case, hunger. Follow these rules every time you have a strong urge to eat or a specific craving.

1. Rate your urge on a scale of one to ten.

2. Repeat this affirmation three times: "Even though I have this craving, I deeply and completely accept myself."

3. Using two fingers on your right hand, tap fifteen to twenty times directly under your right eye. About half an inch to one inch down is perfect. You do not have to tap very hard.

4. Tap fifteen to twenty times directly under the right armpit, approximately three to four inches down.

5. Tap the top of your collarbone fifteen to twenty times. This is located approximately half an inch below the small dip in the front of the neck, and two to three inches to the right on your chest.

6. Find the "gamut spot" on the back of your left hand. This is located between your little finger and your ring finger, approximately one inch below the "V" on the back of your hand. Tap repeatedly on this spot as you do the following:

❑ Keep your eyes open for five seconds.

❑ Close your eyes for five seconds.

❏ Open your eyes for five seconds.

❏ While keeping your head still, move your eyes down to the right and hold for five seconds.

❏ While keeping your head still, move your eyes down to the left and hold for five seconds.

❏ Roll your eyes in a circle to the right.

❏ Roll your eyes in a circle to the left.

❏ Count to five out loud.

❏ Hum a tune out loud for five seconds.

❏ Count to five out loud again.

❏ While keeping your head straight, look down as far as you can and slowly move your eyes upward until you are looking up as high as you can.

7. Slowly take three deep breaths.

8. Ask yourself what your urge is now on a scale of one to ten. If it is gone, you are finished with the process. If it is higher, the same, or only slightly lower than it was before, repeat the process one more time.

This technique should eliminate or dramatically reduce the issue. Sometimes additional patterns and more advanced techniques are required for complete and permanent results. These can be done over the phone with a licensed EFT practitioner who uses special voice recognition technology to determine which points should be tapped and in what sequence. Using this basic technique each time you have an urge or desire will, over time, produce dramatic long-term results.

worked just fine for me, but that may not be the case for everyone. You might consider replacing a portion of your daily meat allowance with an equivalent serving of scrambled, poached or boiled egg for breakfast. Of course, an average-sized egg tends to amount to nearly half of the diet's designated meat portion, so it's a trade-off I made rarely. You could, of course, eat just the egg white, which has about seventeen calories and would use up less of your meat allowance, but doing so was not my preference.

DOWN THE ROAD

As you progress on your journey, you may confront a whole new set of challenges. Just as you encountered and overcame the initial obstacles of the HCG diet, as long as you are prepared, you should be able to handle each and every new bump in the road.

BUILDING IMMUNITY

As you read in Chapter 2, some people develop immunity to HCG. That's why Dr. Simeons' program includes breaks between courses of treatment. Never fear, though. The immunity is not permanent. If you are experiencing extreme hunger or your weight reduction has stalled for a week, you may be becoming immune to HCG. To remedy the problem, stop taking HCG and return to a more normal diet (eating low-calorie, low-fat, low-carb and low-glycemic foods as much as you can tolerate) for at least six weeks. If possible, keep your intake below 1,200 calories a day. When you restart the program, you'll need to fat load again for the first two days before returning to the usual 700-calorie-per-day routine. If necessary, you can repeat these cycles until you reach your goal weight.

You may, of course, decide to take breaks no matter what, which is fine. I chose not to do so, simply because I know myself and was concerned that I might follow one course of treatment, take a break, and then never continue the plan to reach my goal weight. The choice is yours. Be honest with yourself, since no one knows you better.

ADDRESSING THE NEEDS OF YOUR FAMILY

You're on the diet, but your family is not. There is probably not a family in America that wouldn't benefit from a more healthful diet, but you cannot force every member of your household to do what you do. My husband and I created a modus vivendi, or way of living, that worked pretty well.

At dinnertime, I cooked whatever I was going to eat—which was usually chicken or beef, some vegetables and soup or salad—for both of us. I just added an extra carb to the meal for my husband—usually some brown rice or a baked potato. He was wonderfully supportive of my decision to follow the HCG diet, so occasionally when he wanted a chicken curry or spaghetti—foods that were way off my diet—I cooked them just for him with a smile and made sure there were no leftovers to entice me. He doesn't have any excess weight and tends to eat lots of bread and cereal at breakfast time, but those foods are easy for him to prepare, so he usually made his own meal every morning. Obviously, he was on his own again at lunchtime when he was at his workplace.

If you have children, the situation may be a little trickier, but the HCG diet gives you a very good opportunity to get junk food out of your house and feed your kids a more healthful diet that includes celery sticks, carrot sticks, apple slices and popcorn as snacks. The kids' meals can be similar to yours, perhaps with a few added carbs.

I strongly encourage you to enlist the help of your family while you're on this diet. Ask your family members to keep tempting foods out of your home. There's no need to bake cookies, or keep candy or chips around the house. These foods are unreasonably hard to resist, and junk food is simply not good for anybody. You might meet with resistance from your children, but hey, you're the adult and you make the decisions. Your healthful choices will serve them well for the rest of their lives.

Maintaining a Social Life

We all want a social life. It is human nature. But the HCG diet and what most of us consider a normal social life are uneasy partners until you are well grounded in the routine, which takes six weeks or so. If that is all the time you intend to be on the diet, you can just tough it out. Tell your friends what you're doing, ask for their support and stay home as much as possible. Read a good book instead of dining out. Watch a movie on the couch instead of going to a movie theater.

But what if you have a considerable amount of weight to lose and are planning to follow the diet for six months or more, as I did? I work at home, far outside of town, so my social contact is pretty limited. I would never want to become so isolated that I felt like a hermit living in the Himalayas for half a year. Thankfully, I figured out a few ways to maintain a social life while sticking to the HCG diet.

■ **Be Honest.** When you get invited to dinner at a friend's house, you have two options. You can tell your friend about your diet and ask if she would be offended if you brought your own food (and some to share, of course), or you can decline the invitation. I found it was always better to be honest and ask for the support of friends. After all, social occasions are about the company and not really about the food, right?

■ **Get the Home-Field Advantage.** When a friend invites you to a restaurant, invite her to your house instead. This way you have the advantage of controlling the menu. For example, if it's a lunch, serve a salad with chicken and a bowl of soup. Most people are happy with this meal, and so will you be, as it allows you to stay on your weight-loss plan easily. If a guest wants a little something extra, add a piece or two of bread.

■ **Do the Restaurant Research.** If a get-together must take place at a restaurant, things can be a bit tricky. To be honest, I declined these invitations as much as possible. If it is absolutely necessary for you to attend a social function (a spouse's birthday party comes to mind), do a little online research first and look at the restaurant's menu. Many menus have calorie counts and a few even advertise low-calorie meals. Usually the portion sizes will be too large, but you can ask your server to bring a to-go box to the table along with your meal so you can divide your food into appropriate portions. It also helps to carry a diet-friendly serving of your salad dressing of choice in a little bottle to use on these occasions. But, as I've said before, little slips here and there don't spell disaster. Just get back on track as soon as you can.

■ **Weigh Your Options.** The best way to be sociable while on the diet is to suggest activities that do not involve food. I like to play board games with friends. In addition, there are always movie dates, walks, sporting events and even going for coffee (as long as you stick to coffee or tea and can handle the temptation of the baked goods usually offered at coffee houses). When you really think about it, there are all manner of recreational activities to enjoy that will give you social contact without the food problem.

TRAVELING

If you're on the HCG diet for an extended period of time, you may have to fit travel plans into your routine. I found myself dealing with this issue about four months into my diet when I needed to conduct business out of town as well as visit family. How did I handle it? By planning, planning, and planning. My dear friend

Eleanor, a recovering food addict, offered me some helpful ways to get organized at the time. Her major piece of advice: Plan meals in advance and don't get distracted from the plan.

When I traveled by plane, I carried my HCG in my checked luggage. Because the HCG needs to be kept cool, I bundled it with a frozen gel pack and a package of frozen cooked chicken breast. To my delight, everything was still very cold when the plane touched down, despite the fact that more than twelve hours had passed. I also had a bottle of my special salad dressing in my checked luggage, carefully sealed in a plastic bag to prevent leakage.

As for food to eat on the plane, I brought lots of celery sticks, sliced peppers, cherry tomatoes, raw broccoli and a couple of apples in my carry-on. I gave up on the idea of having a salad, since the Transportation Security Administration was following a no-liquid rule at the time, which precluded taking any dressing on board the flight. I suppose vegetable finger foods made more sense, anyway, being less messy.

Once I arrived at my destination, I visited a supermarket and bought some fruit and lettuce to keep in the fridge in my hotel room. My only deviation from the diet was a package of chicken breast from the deli, which I bought when my home-cooked chicken was all gone. When I'm at home, I don't eat deli meats, but this seemed like a logical concession, since I did not have access to cooking facilities while staying at the hotel.

I was able to eat breakfast in my room most days, and could usually escape for lunch and take a break from the intensity of my scheduled business. As for business dinners, which I had to attend over a few nights, I was able to remain on the straight and narrow for all of them. (It helped that California requires calorie counts on menus.) I think my biggest problem was keeping my water intake at the optimal level during the business portion of the trip. My daily calorie count was slightly higher than usual—in the range of about 800 to 900 calories per day.

BEING LAZY

After a few months on the diet, I got a little lazy. With the process firmly in place, I figured the pounds would continue to melt away with little to no effort. The eating plan was pretty much ingrained in me, but, of course, there were occasional lapses. A restaurant meal, a bite of chocolate cake that my husband had brought home, an extra glass of wine at a dinner party—these are all examples of my indiscretions. And what was the result of these indulgences? Not a disaster, just a slowed rate of weight loss. And I don't believe I was any less committed to the HCG diet at the time. I think I simply became too familiar with it. Writing this book actually helped me realize this fact.

During the last week of my first three months on the diet, when I fully expected to reach the halfway point goal of losing fifty pounds, I fell three pounds short of the mark. Did I feel defeated? Like a failure? Not a chance! While the old me might have embraced such negativity, the new me was very proud of every single ounce, and of the fact that I had shed forty-seven pounds of unsightly fat. The shortfall only inspired me to double my efforts and pay closer attention to what I was doing. There was still no free lunch. Two months later, I was back on track, despite experiencing bouts of terrible stress that made the diet difficult and sometimes downright impossible. Once I realized that I'd lost seventy pounds in five months, I felt unstoppable!

FEELING BORED

Let's face it, we are surrounded by advertising on a daily basis. It pushes every sort of sandwich, soft drink and snack right in our faces. We watch television shows that feature families sitting down to dinners that could only be described as banquets. The fact is we live in a commercially driven food-lovers' society. So, what happens when we begin the HCG food regimen? We immediately see it as a very plain diet. To ease into the food shock, I was able to find some fairly creative ways that made life a little more interesting. (Though, there is a part of you that must simply decide to do the diet and not complain.)

My soups not only alleviated the feeling of cold I'd been experiencing, they also added variety to my meals. I figured out how to make a really tasty onion soup that includes onions and garlic that have been caramelized with stevia, all simmered in beef broth. And my chicken soup is essentially a wide variety of vegetables simmered in chicken broth. I sometimes make my soup creamy by blending half of it in a food processor and then stirring the creamy mixture back into the chunky half.

As you know, an occasional bowl of popcorn can be a welcome treat, and, of course, there are endless varieties of tea to enjoy. (Remember, the more liquid you drink, the fuller you fill, so tea can really take the edge off of hunger.) If you don't like tea, there is always lemon or lime juice in water.

As I mentioned earlier, herbs and spices are a huge help, as are simple condiments like mustard (a little added water can make a mustard sauce for your chicken). Even a teaspoon or two of red wine can help bring out the flavor in a piece of sirloin. Perhaps the most unexpected side effect of the HCG diet is that it made me discover my love for simple food. Perhaps I should put out a cookbook one day! Until then, there are many wonderful recipes available online. (See the Resources on page 93.) Ultimately, it has not been difficult to continue eating this way even now that I've reached my goal weight.

WANTING ACKNOWLEDGEMENT

So you've been on the diet for a few weeks and now your clothes are a little bit big on you. You stand in front of the mirror and don't really see a difference quite yet, but your loose pants tell you that the program is working. But then you run into a friend and she doesn't say one word about your weight loss. Nothing! This is a big stumbling block that, like a few of the others, requires a change in mindset. I know I was devastated when, after I lost forty pounds, not a single person said anything about my weight loss unless I pointed it out myself. I knew how much better I looked and how much better I felt, but no one else did.

Thankfully, my husband pointed out two things that should have been obvious to me at the time. The first was that I was still wearing my ridiculously baggy old clothes, which, I erroneously believed, covered up my fat. (In fact, I had begun calling them my "clown clothes" and delighted in pointing out how big they were.) I didn't realize that they were actually hiding my slenderized form. My husband's second point was that it was winter, when we all tend to wear more and bulkier clothes to stay warm. How could I expect the slimmer me to be noticed under all those layers?

I had to be patient, and patience is truly the only advice I can offer for this problem. By the time I had lost close to fifty pounds, I was confident that I would eventually see a friend who would not recognize me. Just a few weeks later, the fantasy came true. Soon after, I bought a very sparkly silver cowgirl belt (for one dollar at a thrift store) and wore it proudly to show off my newly visible waist. It was the first belt I had bought in more than twenty years. Yee-haw! As I approached my goal weight, more and more friends stopped in their tracks and shrieked in disbelief when they finally recognized me. I joked that I was going to have to start wearing a name tag!

Conclusion

It is important to realize that the HCG diet is not about punishment for past behavior. It is about taking control of your life, being an adult, being in charge of what you eat and, ultimately, being in charge of your health and potential for a long life. But the HCG diet is hard work, and hard work deserves a reward. In the past, I probably would have congratulated myself on my effort with a food treat. Those days are gone, but I can still pat myself on the back with a bubble bath, massage, long chat on the phone with a distant friend or evening out to see the latest movie.

I personally found meditation and time alone to be great rewards while on the diet. A little soak in the hot tub is a blessing at the end of the day. I also appreciated the value of assistance. My friend Lydia Belton, a psychotherapist and hypnotherapist who goes by the name Dr. Tranquility, gave me the invaluable gift of weekly hypnotherapy sessions, which allowed me to recognize the way my old mindset had led to an unbalanced relationship with food and my eventual obesity.

Although I have taken the time to tell you how to deal with the obstacles you might encounter while on the HCG diet, truthfully, there is only one rule that will ensure weight loss: Be good to yourself. I eat when I'm stressed and, like everyone else, I encounter stress on a daily basis. Stress can cause disrupt your diet considerably. Recognizing and resisting old thought patterns is a tremendously powerful way to overcome these disruptions. If you slip a little while following the program, don't beat yourself up over it. Pick yourself up, move on and know that you are truly heroic in your endeavor. Beating yourself up only adds to your stress, creating a vicious circle of anxiety. So, again, as much as possible, be good to yourself.

8

Building Self~Esteem

elf-esteem makes all the difference in how you view the world and yourself, as well as how others view you. I grew up hearing the cliché, "It's not what's on the outside that counts, but what's on the inside." To some degree that might be true, but, in the real world, looks definitely count. Appearance plays an important role in business and personal relationships and should not be underestimated. While HCG and caloric restriction help with weight loss, true personal transformation will not occur without an improvement of your self-image. By keeping yourself fit through exercise and maintaining a flattering wardrobe, you will boost your confidence immensely, and confidence is the key to changing not only your measurements but your entire life.

THE IMPORTANCE OF EXERCISE

Most people think that a demanding exercise program is the foundation of any good diet. Most doctors will tell you the same thing, so it must be true, right? Wrong! You'll probably be relieved to

75

know that strenuous exercise is not only absent from the HCG diet, it is also discouraged. In fact, too much exercise could cause your HCG diet to fail. This does not mean, however, that physical fitness isn't an important part of the plan. By toning your body and increasing your stamina, you complete the process that began with weight loss. By getting in shape, you improve yourself inside and out, building the confidence and self-esteem that will help keep the weight off. I know this for a fact because that's what it did for me, as you will read in the following story.

One morning, about four months into the diet, while my neighbor and I were gabbing over the fence, I put my hands on my waist and felt something very strange. There was something hard there under my hands. It actually startled me! It took a second or two for me to realize that this "hard stuff" around my waist was muscle. It was like running into a friend I hadn't seen in a long time, since my waistline had been defined by squishy fat as far back as I could recall. The transformation felt nice and I noticed a sharp rise in confidence immediately.

As you can see, becoming fit helps build self-esteem, which is essential to making your weight loss permanent. But fitness routines must be undertaken in a moderate way while on the HCG program, otherwise you risk compromising your diet. Intense exercise builds appetite and persuades you to take in more calories, which you justify by thinking you've done a good thing by engaging in a rigorous workout. This is a diet buster if there ever was one! In addition, the combination of a low-calorie diet and strenuous exercise can throw your body into starvation mode, causing it to hold on to the weight you're trying to shed by burning muscle instead of fat. Finally, arduous exercise may be too much for your stamina level while on the HCG diet. Your inability to work out in such a manner could possibly act as a source of disappointment, causing you to lose your commitment to the plan altogether.

As both a yoga practitioner and teacher throughout most of my adult life, I am a big proponent of exercise. But for the duration of the HCG diet, your exercise plan should be mild, consisting of twenty to thirty minutes of yoga or light walking, or fifteen minutes of slightly more intense cardiovascular or strength training, no more. Because I believe in the importance of strenuous exercise, I was a little reluctant to give it up for the duration of the HCG diet. But I'm convinced that it is necessary to do so. Now that I can return to my full exercise program, I'll simply do it with more energy and enthusiasm! Maybe I'll even buy a mountain bike to celebrate my new right-sized body.

THE TRANSFORMATIVE POWER OF A NEW WARDROBE

For the first time in decades, clothing is at the forefront of my mind. It seems I was satisfied with couture made by tent manufacturers over the past twenty years, as my family photo album proves. Well, things have changed. "My pants are falling down!" This is by far my favorite complaint these days. You can pretty much assume that you'll go down one size for every twenty pounds lost. Over the course of losing 100 pounds, I went down five dress sizes. Of course, nothing fits!

I garden, take care of my dogs and horses, haul hay and feed, and muck out my barn. Because I also work from home, my wardrobe is always going to consist of jeans, t-shirts and sweatshirts, regardless of my size. Now, however, I wear slightly nicer, more form-fitting jeans and shirts, especially when I go to town and for most social occasions. Although my wardrobe is simple, having clothes that fit well and reveal my new figure gives me a powerful sense of accomplishment and an abundance of self-esteem.

I hoped to update my wardrobe only once during my diet, but that did not turn out to be the case. If you have a considerable amount of weight to lose, as I had, you may need to update your wardrobe two or more times, which can get quite pricey. My budget-minded solution to this issue is to shop at thrift stores and wait until you reach your goal weight to splurge on more expensive new clothes. I picked up four sweaters and a fairly nice pair of jeans one time, spending a total of about forty dollars. When I needed some business clothes to wear to a convention, I was right back at the thrift store, this time to choose a couple of jackets, tops and pants. I spent another forty to fifty dollars and was good to go—except that one of the jackets I'd picked up was actually too big by the time I wore it three weeks later!

I bought a few very nice items of clothing in my final size, which is now a medium, or between a 10 and a 12. I cleaned out my closets, putting my old fat clothes in garbage bags and donating them to a thrift store, or recycling them through my local Freecycle Network group. The act of looking in my closet and removing clothes that no longer fit due to my weight loss always provided me with a major psychological boost. It will do the same for you. And once you see all the empty closet space just begging to be filled, you will feel inspired to create a new wardrobe that reflects not only your new shape but also your newfound confidence.

Conclusion

You will undoubtedly encounter challenges as you take your HCG journey towards your target weight. You'll have some days when you feel great and others when you want to throw in the towel. You'll have some days when you think you could go on eating according to the HCG program forever and others when you obsess endlessly over a now-forbidden favorite food. But once you've built up your self-esteem and confidence, the bad days will be easily overcome.

I have found that becoming physically fit through moderate exercise encourages a positive attitude. When I felt my body getting tighter and noticed fat disappearing from my frame, I became happy and reassured. Replacing my wardrobe with items of clothing that suit my new form also helped to reenergize my efforts. If you pay a little more attention to your appearance, you'll end up looking better than you ever thought you could, I promise. This will inspire you to stick with the diet in times of doubt. When you look good and feel good, you will be less likely to jeopardize your success, which will make you look and feel even better, leading to further success.

In addition to staying positive through exercise and updates to my wardrobe, I made a point not to allow negative thoughts to deter me. Write the following statement on a piece of paper, attach it to your mirror and repeat it aloud several times a day: "I'm doing the HCG diet for me and me alone. I am healthy, strong and capable. I will reach my goal weight and stay there for the rest of my life." Even if it doesn't seem true when you begin, it will before long, I assure you. By the time you finish the diet, you will have reduced your waistline and raised your self-esteem permanently.

9

Keeping the Weight Off

As is the case with any successful diet plan, there comes a time when you reach your ideal weight. Unfortunately, most people start putting the pounds back on almost as soon as they've accomplished their goal. I have met several people who were able to shed their excess weight easily and quickly, but seemed to gain it back just as easily and quickly. I find that this is often the case with people who have only twenty to twenty-five pounds to lose. Perhaps it is because the weight disappears so rapidly that there isn't enough time to permanently adopt new eating patterns or become emotionally invested in self-improvement. In addition, weight loss may occur so fast that the dieter's endocrine system doesn't have time to reset, allowing old metabolic patterns to reemerge.

As you know, HCG reeducates your body to accept its new weight as its natural default, preventing your body from trying to regain the fat it lost. When the diet isn't followed until its completion, the process does not take root permanently.

THE IMPORTANCE OF PHASE THREE

In my experience, greater long-term success is associated with dieters who are on the HCG diet for extended periods of time. Perhaps this is because healthful eating habits become second nature to those who follow the diet for several months, but I suspect there is more at work here. While the change in attitude certainly contributes to success, I think that phase three of the Simeons Protocols is even more important to permanent weight loss. It is this phase that creates a new base weight for your body, preventing weight gain even if you occasionally overindulge. (No, you can't gorge yourself after the diet ends and expect your metabolism to automatically compensate for it.)

When you reach your goal weight and discontinue taking HCG, phase three begins, during which you continue to follow the low-calorie eating plan for three more days and the low-carbohydrate routine for three more weeks. I am told that this is perhaps the most crucial aspect of the diet in regards to avoiding the return of excess pounds. After the first three days, you can increase your caloric intake, including fat (not to an unlimited degree, though!), but must still refrain from eating any carbohydrate-rich foods for three weeks. Specifically, you cannot eat sugar, rice, pasta, bread (except the very small amount you ate when you were restricting your meals to 700 calories a day) or potatoes. While you can increase your fat consumption, you must avoid these carbs. Doing so allows you to reach a new and permanent set point for your metabolic rate.

I recommend you weigh yourself every morning during this period. A weight gain of more than two pounds in one day should be cause for alarm. It triggers a protocol that requires you to eat only a large steak and an apple or tomato in one twenty-four-hour period, which should help establish the metabolic reset properly, provided you resume the low-carbohydrate phase. This makes sense to me, and I faithfully followed this recommendation during my own phase three. Why go through all this work only to mess it up at the end, right? I actually had a conversation with someone who went through the entire process only to regain the weight afterwards. Upon questioning, she admitted that she had not thought the final phase necessary and so had not completed it.

Conclusion

"Yes, in the interest of long-term weight control, I can tough it out for three more weeks and not dive into a plate of spaghetti." This is the attitude you must adopt if you truly wish to transform your life. Phase three is probably the most important part of the entire HCG program. When you're all the way through the plan, you can go back to eating normally. Of course, "eating normally" won't mean what it meant before the HCG diet. Not only will you have reset your default weight level, you will have reinvented your relationship with food, and it will be easy to stay committed to a healthful meal plan your whole life long.

When I reached my goal weight, I found that 1600 calories of food per day allowed me to maintain it. I didn't fantasize about adding pizza or chocolate cake. Initially, it was a little difficult to raise my caloric intake by more than double, to be honest. (I even added some low-fat cheese and a baked potato to my diet.) Now that I have shed all my unwanted fat, I am confident I will be able to stay slim and healthy for the rest of my life. I know you will be able to do the same.

Conclusion

I believe that this simplified version of the HCG diet is a panacea for the obesity epidemic of the twenty-first century. Millions of people are overweight and millions have attempted to get rid of unwanted fat without permanent success. Weight-loss programs including the Atkins Diet, the South Beach Diet, the Grapefruit Diet, Jenny Craig, Nutrisystem and Weight Watchers—not to mention all the stranger, arguably unhealthful diets out there—have had little effect on the problem and are almost never associated with stories of long-term weight-loss accomplishments.

Now millions of overweight, obese and morbidly obese people can find hope in the Super Simple HCG Diet. By following this fat-busting regimen, those who wish to shed extra pounds and attain an optimal weight now have the opportunity to do so safely and painlessly. The benefits of this plan are impressive and can add many healthy years to your life. Best of all, the HCG diet has very few contraindications, so it can be effective for almost anyone.

I hope this book has been not only helpful but also inspirational. I would truly love to see you begin your journey towards a new body, attitude and life. The first step is now yours to take. If there are missteps, so be it. Pick yourself up, dust yourself off and begin again. If you follow the simple guidelines outlined in this book, I have no doubt you'll succeed.

Calorie Counts

The following table lists the calorie count of each "must eat" and allowable food mentioned in Chapter 3 according to portion size.

FOOD	PORTION SIZE	CALORIES
alfalfa sprouts	1/2 cup	5
apples	1 medium-sized apple	72
artichokes	1 medium-sized artichoke	64
asparagus	1/2 cup	20
beef, flank	3 1/2 ounces	192
beef, ground round	3 1/2 ounces	150
beef, sirloin	3 1/2 ounces	160
beef, tenderloin	3 1/2 ounces	200
beef, top round	3 1/2 ounces	166
beef, tri-tip	3 1/2 ounces	260
beer, low-calorie	12 ounces	100
beet greens	1/2 cup	20
bell peppers, green	1/2 cup	15
bell peppers, red	1/2 cup	23
bell peppers, yellow	1/2 cup	25

FOOD	PORTION SIZE	CALORIES
blackberries	1/2 cup	31
blueberries	1/2 cup	42
broccoli	1/2 cup	27
cabbage	1/2 cup	11
cantaloupe	1/2 cup	30
cauliflower	1/2 cup	14
cherries	1/2 cup	37
chicken breast, boneless and skinless	3 1/2 ounces	97
clementines	1 medium-sized clementine	35
collard greens	1/2 cup	25
distilled spirits, brandy	1 1/2 ounces	65
distilled spirits, gin	1 1/2 ounces	65
distilled spirits, rum	1 1/2 ounces	65
distilled spirits, vodka	1 1/2 ounces	65
distilled spirits, whiskey	1 1/2 ounces	65
fish, cod	3 1/2 ounces	104
fish, crab	3 1/2 ounces	96
fish, flounder	3 1/2 ounces	116
fish, haddock	3 1/2 ounces	110
fish, halibut	3 1/2 ounces	138

FOOD	PORTION SIZE	CALORIES
fish, lobster	3 1/2 ounces	89
fish, sea bass	3 1/2 ounces	122
fish, shrimp	3 1/2 ounces	98
fish, tilapia	3 1/2 ounces	128
grapefruit	1/2 cup	49
grapes	1/2 cup	31
green beans	1/2 cup	22
honeydew melon	1/2 cup	32
kale	1/2 cup	18
Mandarin oranges	1/2 cup	75
multigrain sandwich rounds	1 round	100
multigrain tortillas	1 tortilla	100
mushrooms	1/2 cup	11
mustard greens	1/2 cup	10
nectarines	1 medium-sized nectarine	62
peaches	1 medium-sized peach	38
pears	1 medium-sized pear	96
popcorn (air-popped) without butter	1/2 cup	16
pork loin	3 1/2 ounces	192

FOOD	PORTION SIZE	CALORIES
raspberries	1/2 cup	32
red radishes	1/2 cup	10
salad greens	1/2 cup	5
spinach	1/2 cup	4
squash	1 medium-sized squash	31
strawberries	1/2 cup	25
Swiss chard	1/2 cup	4
tomatoes	1 medium-sized tomato	26
turkey breast, bone-less and skinless	3 1/2 ounces	88
watermelon	1/2 cup	23
whole grain bread, non-fat	1 slice	100
whole grain flat bread	1 piece	100
wine, dry, red	4 ounces	85
wine, dry, white	4 ounces	91

Glycemic Index Chart

The following chart includes the glycemic index ranges of the "must eat" and allowable foods detailed in Chapter 3. Foods that do not cause a significantly measurable rise in blood glucose levels, such as lean meats, have been excluded.

Food	Low GI (0–55)	Mid GI (56–69)	High GI (70–100)
apples	▓		
artichokes	▓		
asparagus	▓		
beet greens	▓		
blackberries	▓		
blueberries	▓		
broccoli	▓		
Brussels sprouts	▓		
cabbage	▓		
cantaloupe		▓	
cauliflower	▓		
celery	▓		
cherries	▓		
clementines			▓
collard greens	▓		
dill pickles	▓		
garlic	▓		
grapefruit	▓		
grapes	▓		
green beans	▓		

Food	Low GI (0–55)	Mid GI (56–69)	High GI (70–100)
honeydew melon			▨
kale	▨		
Mandarin oranges	▨		
multigrain sandwich rounds	▨		
multigrain tortillas	▨		
mushrooms	▨		
mustard greens	▨		
nectarines		▨	
onions	▨		
peaches	▨		
pears	▨		
peppers (all varieties)	▨		
popcorn (air-popped) without butter			▨
raspberries	▨		
red radishes	▨		
salad greens	▨		
spinach	▨		
sprouts	▨		
squash	▨		
strawberries	▨		
Swiss chard	▨		
tomatoes	▨		
watermelon			▨
whole grain bread, non-fat	▨		
whole grain flat bread	▨		

Resources

Because there are a great number of supplement sellers that offer oral HCG drops of questionable quality, it is important to find a few reputable manufacturers or distributors of effective HCG drops, which are detailed here. This section also provides resources to help you reduce the anxiety and other psychological difficulties that often crop up as you follow the HCG diet program. Finally, there are a number of websites listed below, which can help you learn about the original HCG diet, find a physician to guide you through the program, and remain aware of the nutritional value of the food you eat once the diet is over.

ORAL HCG DISTRIBUTORS

AnuMed-Intl

Phone: (888) 921-3880

Website: www.anumed-intl.com

AnuMed-Intl is an online store that focuses on homeopathic medicine and other dietary supplements. They offer a version of HCG drops that comes with a menu book to help you lose weight.

Tahoma Clinic Dispensary

801 SW 16th, Suite 125

Renton, WA 98057

Phone: (425) 264-0051

Website: www.tahomadispensary.com

The Tahoma Clinic features a variety of products related to alternative health care, including organic foods, informational publications, and natural supplements such as HCG drops. The formulas for its supplements are chosen and tested by the clinic's own doctors and staff.

Tango Advanced Nutrition

1311 Church Street

San Francisco, CA 94114

Phone: (866) 778-2646, ext. 1

Website: www.puretango.com

Tango Advanced Nutrition is the distributor of a number of dietary supplements, many of which have been designed by leading Chinese herbal researchers. They also sell HCG drops that feature a specific blend of amino acids to support blood flow and increase energy.

PSYCHOLOGICAL AIDS

Kripalu Center for Yoga and Health

PO Box 309

Stockbridge, MA 01262

Phone: (866) 200-5203

Website: www.kripalu.org

Kripalu Center for Yoga & Health is a nonprofit educational organization focused on the spiritual and scientific aspects of yoga. It seeks to teach others about the meditative and health-giving properties of the practice. In addition to offering training programs and retreats, the center can help you find a Kripalu practitioner in your area.

The Tapping Solution

Website: www.thetappingsolution.com

This website is dedicated to the documentary film of the same name as well as an accompanying book, both of which seek to explain and teach the Emotional Freedom Technique for relief of anxiety. Both of these products can be purchased through the website.

HELPFUL WEBSITES

Freedieting

Website: www.freedieting.com/tools/calorie_calculator.htm

Using your weight, height, age, gender, and level of physical activity, this website calculates the amount of daily calories required to maintain your present weight. It can be a very helpful source of information once you've reached your goal.

HCG Diet Info

Website: www.hcgdietinfo.com

This website features Dr. Simeons' book, Pounds and Inches, *in its entirety for you to read free of charge. In addition to a wealth of other HCG-related information, it also includes HCG diet-friendly recipes, which can be very helpful when you're trying to keep your meal plan interesting.*

HCG Provider Directory

Website: www.hcgproviderdirectory.com

This website lists the clinics and doctors throughout the country that offer the HCG diet. It can be helpful when looking for an HCG provider in your area.

Mendosa

Website: www.mendosa.com/gilists.htm

Run by freelance medical writer David Mendosa, this website offers a wealth of resources for people living with diabetes, including a comprehensive list of the glycemic load values of thousands of foods.

Mike's Calorie and Fat Gram Chart for 1,000 Foods

Website: www.caloriecountercharts.com

This website lists one thousand foods according to their calorie count, fat content, cholesterol content, protein content, and carbohydrate content. It can be a powerful resource in weight management.

Diet Diary

When you are on a 700-calorie-per-day program such as the one outlined in the Super Simple HCG Diet, it is tremendously important to keep track of the foods you eat. Food portions and their according calorie counts are vital pieces of information to record and use as a reference, particularly when you are starting a new daily meal plan. The following diet diary includes a daily food log that enables you to monitor your food consumption at breakfast, lunch, dinner, and even snack time, helping to reveal the way in which you divide your "must eat" and allowable foods throughout the day. Simply measure your food, determine the calorie count of each portion by referencing "Calorie Counts" on page 87, and mark the information in the appropriate box. The log also includes a way to chart your water intake. All you have to do is cross out one cup graphic for each eight-ounce glass of water you drink.

While an accurate account of your food intake is a fundamental part of a successful diet, your hunger levels and feelings about your experience may be just as crucial. This regimen will likely be a big adjustment to your lifestyle and can initially cause emotions to run wild. Writing them down is a good way to keep them in check, which is why this section also includes journal pages. You can also use this space to note your exercise habits and any stress management techniques you may employ. If you feel the need to continue using a diary for a longer time than the two-week period provided, simply do so in a separate notebook. Whatever gets you to your target weight!

Your Daily Food Log   DATE _____

	FOOD	PORTION	CALORIES	H₂O
BREAKFAST				$\square$
				$\square$
				$\square$

						H₂O
SNACK						$\square$
						$\square$

	FOOD	PORTION	CALORIES	H₂O
LUNCH				$\square$
				$\square$
				$\square$

						H₂O
SNACK						$\square$
						$\square$

	FOOD	PORTION	CALORIES	H₂O
DINNER				$\square$
				$\square$
				$\square$

Your Journal

Breakfast

Hunger Level: ❑ **Extreme** ❑ **Moderate** ❑ **Low**

Feelings:

_____

_____

_____

_____

_____

Lunch

Hunger Level: ❑ **Extreme** ❑ **Moderate** ❑ **Low**

Feelings:

_____

_____

_____

_____

_____

Dinner

Hunger Level: ❑ **Extreme** ❑ **Moderate** ❑ **Low**

Feelings:

_____

_____

_____

_____

_____

Your Daily Food Log   DATE _____

	FOOD	PORTION	CALORIES	H₂O
BREAKFAST				

						H₂O
SNACK						

	FOOD	PORTION	CALORIES	H₂O
LUNCH				

						H₂O
SNACK						

	FOOD	PORTION	CALORIES	H₂O
DINNER				

100

Your Journal

Breakfast

Hunger Level: ❏ Extreme   ❏ Moderate   ❏ Low

Feelings:
_____

_____

_____

_____

Lunch

Hunger Level: ❏ Extreme   ❏ Moderate   ❏ Low

Feelings:
_____

_____

_____

_____

Dinner

Hunger Level: ❏ Extreme   ❏ Moderate   ❏ Low

Feelings:
_____

_____

_____

_____

Your Daily Food Log   DATE _____

BREAKFAST	FOOD	PORTION	CALORIES	H₂O

SNACK						H₂O

LUNCH	FOOD	PORTION	CALORIES	H₂O

SNACK						H₂O

DINNER	FOOD	PORTION	CALORIES	H₂O

102

Your Journal

Breakfast

Hunger Level: ❏ **Extreme**   ❏ **Moderate**   ❏ **Low**

Feelings: _____

_____

_____

_____

_____

Lunch

Hunger Level: ❏ **Extreme**   ❏ **Moderate**   ❏ **Low**

Feelings: _____

_____

_____

_____

_____

Dinner

Hunger Level: ❏ **Extreme**   ❏ **Moderate**   ❏ **Low**

Feelings: _____

_____

_____

_____

_____

Your Daily Food Log   DATE _____

	FOOD	PORTION	CALORIES	H₂O
BREAKFAST				

						H₂O
SNACK						

	FOOD	PORTION	CALORIES	H₂O
LUNCH				

						H₂O
SNACK						

	FOOD	PORTION	CALORIES	H₂O
DINNER				

Your Journal

Breakfast

Hunger Level: ❏ Extreme   ❏ Moderate   ❏ Low

Feelings: _____

_____

_____

_____

_____

Lunch

Hunger Level: ❏ Extreme   ❏ Moderate   ❏ Low

Feelings: _____

_____

_____

_____

_____

Dinner

Hunger Level: ❏ Extreme   ❏ Moderate   ❏ Low

Feelings: _____

_____

_____

_____

_____

Your Daily Food Log   DATE _____

	FOOD	PORTION	CALORIES	H₂O
BREAKFAST				

						H₂O
SNACK						

	FOOD	PORTION	CALORIES	H₂O
LUNCH				

						H₂O
SNACK						

	FOOD	PORTION	CALORIES	H₂O
DINNER				

Your Journal

Breakfast

Hunger Level: ❑ Extreme   ❑ Moderate   ❑ Low

Feelings:
_____
_____
_____
_____
_____

Lunch

Hunger Level: ❑ Extreme   ❑ Moderate   ❑ Low

Feelings:
_____
_____
_____
_____
_____

Dinner

Hunger Level: ❑ Extreme   ❑ Moderate   ❑ Low

Feelings:
_____
_____
_____
_____
_____

Your Daily Food Log   DATE _____

	FOOD	PORTION	CALORIES	H₂O
BREAKFAST				$\square$
				$\square$
				$\square$

							H₂O
SNACK							$\square$
							$\square$

	FOOD	PORTION	CALORIES	H₂O
LUNCH				$\square$
				$\square$
				$\square$

							H₂O
SNACK							$\square$
							$\square$

	FOOD	PORTION	CALORIES	H₂O
DINNER				$\square$
				$\square$
				$\square$

Your Journal

Breakfast

Hunger Level: ❑ Extreme ❑ Moderate ❑ Low

Feelings:

_____

_____

_____

_____

Lunch

Hunger Level: ❑ Extreme ❑ Moderate ❑ Low

Feelings:

_____

_____

_____

_____

Dinner

Hunger Level: ❑ Extreme ❑ Moderate ❑ Low

Feelings:

_____

_____

_____

_____

Your Daily Food Log   DATE _____

	FOOD	PORTION	CALORIES	H₂O
BREAKFAST				

						H₂O
SNACK						

	FOOD	PORTION	CALORIES	H₂O
LUNCH				

						H₂O
SNACK						

	FOOD	PORTION	CALORIES	H₂O
DINNER				

Your Journal

Breakfast

Hunger Level: ❑ **Extreme** ❑ **Moderate** ❑ **Low**

Feelings: _____

_____

_____

_____

_____

Lunch

Hunger Level: ❑ **Extreme** ❑ **Moderate** ❑ **Low**

Feelings: _____

_____

_____

_____

_____

Dinner

Hunger Level: ❑ **Extreme** ❑ **Moderate** ❑ **Low**

Feelings: _____

_____

_____

_____

_____

Your Daily Food Log   DATE _____

BREAKFAST	FOOD	PORTION	CALORIES	H₂O
				▽
				▽
				▽

SNACK						H₂O
						▽
						▽

LUNCH	FOOD	PORTION	CALORIES	H₂O
				▽
				▽
				▽

SNACK						H₂O
						▽
						▽

DINNER	FOOD	PORTION	CALORIES	H₂O
				▽
				▽
				▽

Your Journal

Breakfast

Hunger Level: ❏ Extreme   ❏ Moderate   ❏ Low

Feelings: _____

_____

_____

_____

_____

Lunch

Hunger Level: ❏ Extreme   ❏ Moderate   ❏ Low

Feelings: _____

_____

_____

_____

_____

Dinner

Hunger Level: ❏ Extreme   ❏ Moderate   ❏ Low

Feelings: _____

_____

_____

_____

_____

Your Daily Food Log   DATE _____

	FOOD	PORTION	CALORIES	H₂O
BREAKFAST				

SNACK						

	FOOD	PORTION	CALORIES	H₂O
LUNCH				

SNACK						

	FOOD	PORTION	CALORIES	H₂O
DINNER				

Your Journal

Breakfast

Hunger Level: ❏ Extreme   ❏ Moderate   ❏ Low

Feelings: _____

_____

_____

_____

_____

Lunch

Hunger Level: ❏ Extreme   ❏ Moderate   ❏ Low

Feelings: _____

_____

_____

_____

_____

Dinner

Hunger Level: ❏ Extreme   ❏ Moderate   ❏ Low

Feelings: _____

_____

_____

_____

Your Daily Food Log   DATE _____

BREAKFAST	FOOD	PORTION	CALORIES	H₂O
				$\square$
				$\square$
				$\square$

SNACK						H₂O
						$\square$
						$\square$

LUNCH	FOOD	PORTION	CALORIES	H₂O
				$\square$
				$\square$
				$\square$

SNACK						H₂O
						$\square$
						$\square$

DINNER	FOOD	PORTION	CALORIES	H₂O
				$\square$
				$\square$
				$\square$

Your Journal

Breakfast

Hunger Level: ❏ Extreme ❏ Moderate ❏ Low

Feelings: _____

_____

_____

_____

_____

Lunch

Hunger Level: ❏ Extreme ❏ Moderate ❏ Low

Feelings: _____

_____

_____

_____

_____

Dinner

Hunger Level: ❏ Extreme ❏ Moderate ❏ Low

Feelings: _____

_____

_____

_____

_____

Your Daily Food Log   DATE _____

	FOOD	PORTION	CALORIES	H₂O
BREAKFAST				

						H₂O
SNACK						

	FOOD	PORTION	CALORIES	H₂O
LUNCH				

						H₂O
SNACK						

	FOOD	PORTION	CALORIES	H₂O
DINNER				

Your Journal

Breakfast

Hunger Level: ❑ **Extreme** ❑ **Moderate** ❑ **Low**

Feelings: _____

_____

_____

_____

_____

Lunch

Hunger Level: ❑ **Extreme** ❑ **Moderate** ❑ **Low**

Feelings: _____

_____

_____

_____

_____

Dinner

Hunger Level: ❑ **Extreme** ❑ **Moderate** ❑ **Low**

Feelings: _____

_____

_____

_____

_____

Your Daily Food Log   DATE _____

	FOOD	PORTION	CALORIES	H₂O
BREAKFAST				

						H₂O
SNACK						

	FOOD	PORTION	CALORIES	H₂O
LUNCH				

						H₂O
SNACK						

	FOOD	PORTION	CALORIES	H₂O
DINNER				

Your Journal

Breakfast

Hunger Level: ❏ Extreme   ❏ Moderate   ❏ Low

Feelings:
_____

_____

_____

_____

Lunch

Hunger Level: ❏ Extreme   ❏ Moderate   ❏ Low

Feelings:
_____

_____

_____

_____

Dinner

Hunger Level: ❏ Extreme   ❏ Moderate   ❏ Low

Feelings:
_____

_____

_____

_____

Your Daily Food Log   DATE _____

	FOOD	PORTION	CALORIES	H₂O
BREAKFAST				⬚
				⬚
				⬚

					H₂O
SNACK					⬚
					⬚

	FOOD	PORTION	CALORIES	H₂O
LUNCH				⬚
				⬚
				⬚

					H₂O
SNACK					⬚
					⬚

	FOOD	PORTION	CALORIES	H₂O
DINNER				⬚
				⬚
				⬚

Your Journal

Breakfast

Hunger Level: ❑ **Extreme**   ❑ **Moderate**   ❑ **Low**

Feelings: _____

_____

_____

_____

_____

Lunch

Hunger Level: ❑ **Extreme**   ❑ **Moderate**   ❑ **Low**

Feelings: _____

_____

_____

_____

_____

Dinner

Hunger Level: ❑ **Extreme**   ❑ **Moderate**   ❑ **Low**

Feelings: _____

_____

_____

_____

_____

Your Daily Food Log   DATE _____

	FOOD	PORTION	CALORIES	H₂O
BREAKFAST				

						H₂O
SNACK						

	FOOD	PORTION	CALORIES	H₂O
LUNCH				

						H₂O
SNACK						

	FOOD	PORTION	CALORIES	H₂O
DINNER				

124

Your Journal

Breakfast

Hunger Level: ❏ Extreme   ❏ Moderate   ❏ Low

Feelings:

_____

_____

_____

_____

_____

Lunch

Hunger Level: ❏ Extreme   ❏ Moderate   ❏ Low

Feelings:

_____

_____

_____

_____

_____

Dinner

Hunger Level: ❏ Extreme   ❏ Moderate   ❏ Low

Feelings:

_____

_____

_____

_____

_____

About the Author

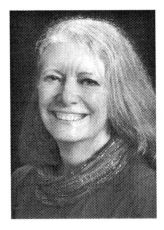

Kathleen Barnes is the author, coauthor, or editor of over a dozen natural health books, including 8 Weeks to Vibrant Health and The Calcium Lie. She enjoyed an early career in newspapers as well as a ten-year stint as a foreign correspondent in Asia and Africa for ABC and CNN before returning to the United States to work in the field of health. For six years, Kathleen wrote the weekly natural health column for Woman's World magazine, and has been a part of the effort to raise public awareness of the subject of natural health for more than thirty years, as both a writer and yoga teacher.

Her passion for wellness and sustainable living has its roots in the early days of the natural health movement. She became a certified Kripalu Yoga teacher in the early 1970s--a time when yoga was still deemed "weird." Although many of the natural healing methods discussed in her writings were considered fringe science at the time, a large number of these formerly ridiculed practices have now been scientifically validated, embraced by mainstream medicine, and widely accepted by society.

After entering menopause at an early age, Kathleen began to put on weight, as so many women do during this transition. Over the course of twenty years, she found herself 100 pounds overweight. While the excess fat did not trigger diabetes, heart disease, or any other serious health condition, it did affect her mobility and aged her prematurely. It also had a profound effect on her self-esteem, in part because her profession and lifestyle were centered on healthful living. She tried over a dozen different diets without success before discovering, modifying, and adopting the HCG diet, which changed everything. Kathleen's version of the HCG diet allowed her to drop 100 pounds and reach a healthful weight in an astounding nine-month period, enhancing her self-esteem and changing her life in more ways than she ever could have imagined.

Kathleen currently lives in rural North Carolina with her husband, Joe, where the two of them enjoy riding their horses and tending their garden.

Index

American Medical Association (AMA), 20

B vitamins, 20–21
Bacteriostatic water, 42
BCM-95, 21
Biological feminization, 56
Biotin, 21. *See also* B vitamins.
Binging. *See* Fat binge.
Blood levels, testing, 45
BMI. *See* Body Mass Index.
Body Mass Index (BMI), 50–51
    chart for, 51
Boredom, 71–72
Boyer, Frankie, 6
Bread. *See* Carbohydrates; "Must eat" bread.
Breakfast, 63, 65
    and Simeons Protocols, 13
Building immunity to HCG, 24, 66–67

Carbohydrates, 16. *See also* "Must eat" bread.
Cass, Hyla, 8
Challenges of the HCG diet. *See* Boredom; Breakfast; Building immunity to HCG; Detoxification; Family needs, addressing; Fear of failure; Feeling cold; Hunger pangs; Laziness; Maintaining a social life; Traveling; Weight-loss, acknowledgment of.
Children, 67
Coffee, 16–17
Cooking methods, 39
Craig, Gary, 64
Cravings, stopping. *See* Emotional Freedom Technique.
Criticism, 24–26
Curcumin, 21

Detoxification, 62
DHA. *See* Docosahexaenoic acid.
Diet
    challenges of. *See* Challenges
        of the HCG diet.
    decision to start, 6–9
    500-calorie versus 700-calorie,
        7, 14–15, 28
    preparations for, 52–53
    setting a starting date for,
        49–50
    taking breaks on, 24, 66
    See also Simeons Protocols.
Dietary supplements. *See*
    Supplements.
Docosahexaenoic acid (DHA), 21
Doctors
    consulting, 44–45
    finding, 46
Dry brushing, 18

Eicosapentaneoic acid (EPA), 21
Eisenstein, Mayer, 23, 55
Emotional Freedom Technique, 62
    using the, 64–65
Endocrine system, 12
EPA. *See* Eicosapentaneoic acid.
Exercise, 75–77

Family needs, addressing, 67–68
Fat binge, 28–29
Fear of failure, 62–63
Feeling cold, 63
Fertility. *See* Pregnancy and the
    HCG diet.

Fish oil, 21–22
Food
    binge. *See* Fat binge.
    cooking, 39
    cravings for, stopping. *See*
        Emotional Freedom
        Technique.
    forbidden, 37–38
    indulgences, 35–36
    measuring, 29–30
    organic. *See* Organic food.
    required. *See* "Must eat" bread;
        "Must eat" fruit; "Must eat"
        meat; "Must eat"   veggies.
    shopping for, 38–39
    unlimited. *See* Unlimited
        foods.
    See also Carbohydrates; Coffee;
        Meat; Salad dressing; Soup;
        Vegetables.
Food journal, 53
Food scales, 29
Freecycle Network, 78
Fruit. *See* "Must eat" fruit.

Gamut spot, 64
Glycemic index, 15, 30–31
Glycemic load, 30–31

HCG
    about, 7, 12
    building immunity to, 24,
        66–67
    and men. *See* Men and the
        HCG diet.

and pregnancy, 56–57
taking by injection, 41–43
taking by oral drops, 43–44
and women. *See* Women and
the HCG diet.
Herbs. *See* Spices and herbs.
Human chorionic gonadotropin
(HCG). *See* HCG.
Hunger pangs, 62
stopping. *See* Emotional
Freedom Technique.
Hypothalamus, 12

Immunity, to HCG. *See* Building
immunity to HCG.
Injections of HCG, 41–43
Iodine. *See* Potassium iodide.

Kripalu yoga, 63

Laziness, 71
Lidocaine, 42

Magnesium, 22
Makeup, use of, 13
Maintaining a social life, 68–69
Massages, 18
Measuring your food, 29–30
Meat, 17. *See also* "Must eat"
meat.
Medical conditions, 45
Meditation, 63
Men and the HCG diet
common questions about,
56–57

success story about, 57–58
and tips for success, 58–59
Menstruation. *See* Women and
HCG diet.
Multivitamins, 22
"Must eat" bread, 34
"Must eat" fruit, 33
"Must eat" meat, 33–34
"Must eat" veggies, 32

Omega-3 fatty acids, 21
Oral HCG drops, 43–44
Organic food, 38–39

Physical fitness. *See* Exercise.
Physicians. *See* Doctors.
Potassium, 22
Potassium iodide, 22
Pounds and Inches (Simeons),
7, 12, 25
Pregnancy and HCG, 56–57

Restaurants, eating at, 69

Salad dressing, 17–18
Scales, food, 29
Self-esteem, building. *See*
Exercise; Wardrobe,
updating;
Simeons, A.T.W., 6, 11–12
Simeons' HCG diet. *See*
Simeons Protocols.
Simeons Protocols
about, 7
guidelines for, 13

phases of, 12--13, 82
simplified version of. *See*
 Carbohydrates; Coffee;
 Meat; "Must eat" bread;
 "Must eat" fruit; "Must eat"
 meat; "Must eat" veggies;
 Salad dressing; Skin creams;
 Soup; Spices and herbs;
 Supplements; Vegetables;
 Unlimited foods.
and taking breaks, 24
Skin creams, 18
Socializing. *See* Maintaining a
 social life.
Soup, 18–19
Spices and herbs, 19–20
Starting the diet. *See*Diet,
 setting a starting date for.
Stevia, 37
Supplements, 20–23
Sweeteners, 37

Tapping technique. *See*
 Emotional Freedom
 Technique.

Target weight, setting, 50–52.
Traveling, 69–70
Turmeric. *See* Curcumin.

Unlimited foods, 34–35

Vegetables, 23. *See also* "Must
 eat" veggies.
Vitamin D, 23

Wardrobe, updating, 77–78
Water
 bacteriostatic, 42
 required intake of, 31
Weighing
 your food. *See* Food scales.
 yourself, 82
Weight loss
 acknowledgement of, 72–73
 in men versus women, 55–56
 maintaining, 81–83
Women and HCG diet, 47. *See
 also* Pregnancy and HCG.

Yoga, Kripalu. *See* Kripalu yoga.

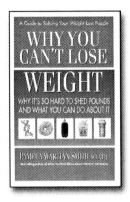

WHY YOU CAN'T LOSE WEIGHT
Why It's So Hard to Shed Pounds and What You Can Do About It
Pamela Wartian Smith, MD, MPH

If you have tried diet after diet without shedding pounds, it may not be your fault. In this revolutionary book, Dr. Pamela Smith discusses the eighteen most common reasons why you can't lose weight, and guides you in overcoming the obstacles that stand between you and a trimmer body.

If you've been frustrated by one-size-fits-all diet plans, it's time to learn what's really keeping you from reaching your goal. With *Why You Can't Lose Weight,* you'll discover how to lose weight and enjoy radiant health.

$16.95 US • 256 pages • 6 x 9-inch quality paperback • ISBN 978-0-7570-0312-7

BITE IT & WRITE IT!
A Guide to Keeping Track of What You Eat & Drink
Stacie Castle, RD, Robyn Cotler, RD, Marni Schefter, RD, and Shana Shapiro, RD

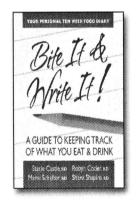

Professionals know that keeping track of what you eat and drink is the most effective way to improve your dietary habits. Designed by nutritionists who have successfully used this system in their practices, *Bite It & Write It!* combines a structured food journal with an easy-to-follow nutrition guide.

Bite It & Write It! presents ten health goals—one for each week of the journal—and lets you record your daily food consumption as you work toward your objective. To help you along the way, the authors supply a wealth of nutritional information that will empower you to change the way you think about food and make a new commitment to improving your health. With this guide, you can track your calories, carbs, sodium, and water; record exercise; learn how to plan and prepare meals; and navigate restaurant menus without blowing your diet.

$7.95 US • 192 pages • 4 x 7-inch mass paperback • ISBN 978-0-7570-0343-1

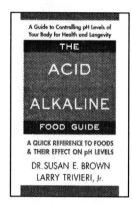

A Guide to Controlling pH Levels of Your Body for Health and Longevity

THE ACID ALKALINE FOOD GUIDE

A QUICK REFERENCE TO FOODS & THEIR EFFECT ON pH LEVELS

DR. SUSAN E. BROWN LARRY TRIVIERI, Jr.

THE ACID-ALKALINE FOOD GUIDE

A Quick Reference to Foods & Their Effect on pH Levels

Dr. Susan E. Brown and Larry Trivieri, Jr.

In the last few years, researchers around the world have reported the importance of acid-alkaline balance to good health. While thousands of people are trying to balance their body's pH level, until now, they have had to rely on guides containing only a small number of foods. *The Acid-Alkaline Food Guide* is a complete resource for people who want to widen their food choices.

The book begins by explaining how the acid-alkaline environment of the body is influenced by foods. It then presents a list of thousands of foods—single foods, combination foods, and even fast foods—and their acid-alkaline effects. *The Acid-Alkaline Food Guide* will quickly become the resource you turn to at home, in restaurants, and whenever you want to select a food that can help you reach your health and dietary goals.

$7.95 • 208 pages • 4 x 7-inch mass paperback • ISBN 978-0-7570-0280-9

GLYCEMIC INDEX FOOD GUIDE

For Weight Loss, Cardiovascular Health, Diabetic Management, and Maximum Energy

Dr. Shari Lieberman

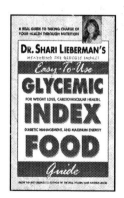

A REAL GUIDE TO TAKING CHARGE OF YOUR HEALTH THROUGH NUTRITION

DR. SHARI LIEBERMAN'S

MEASURING THE GLUCOSE IMPACT

Easy-To-Use

GLYCEMIC

FOR WEIGHT LOSS, CARDIOVASCULAR HEALTH,

INDEX

DIABETIC MANAGEMENT, AND MAXIMUM ENERGY

FOOD

Guide

By indicating how quickly a given food triggers a rise in blood sugar, the glycemic index (GI) enables you to choose foods that can help you easily manage various conditions and improve your overall health. Designed as an easy-to-use guide to the glycemic index, this book first answers commonly asked questions, to ensure that you truly understand the GI and know how to use it. It then provides both the glycemic index and the glycemic load for hundreds of foods and beverages.

$7.95 • 160 pages • 4 x 7-inch mass paperback • ISBN 978-0-7570-0245-8

SUICIDE BY SUGAR
A Startling Look at Our #1 National Addiction
Nancy Appleton, PhD, and G.N. Jacobs

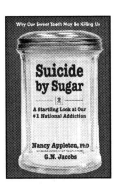

It is a dangerous, addictive white powder that can be found in abundance throughout this country. It is not illegal. In fact, it is available near playgrounds, schools, and vacation spots, and once we are hooked on it, the cravings can be overwhelming. This white substance of abuse is sugar.

Over two decades ago, Nancy Appleton's *Lick the Sugar Habit* exposed the dangers of America's high-sugar diet. Now, *Suicide by Sugar* presents a broader view of the problems caused by our favorite ingredient. The authors offer startling facts linking a range of disorders—from dementia to obesity—to our growing sugar addiction. *Suicide by Sugar* shines a bright light on our nation's addiction and helps us begin the journey toward health.

$15.95 • 192 pages • 6 x 9-inch quality paperback • ISBN 978-0-7570-0306-6

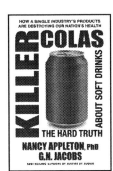

KILLER COLAS
The Hard Truth About Soft Drinks
Nancy Appleton, PhD, and G.N. Jacobs

It's as American as fast foods. So why are people saying all those nasty things about soft drinks? The answer is simple: They're true. In *Killer Colas,* Dr. Nancy Appleton and G.N. Jacobs provide a startling picture of a giant industry hell-bent on destroying our country's health.

Over the last few decades, the sale of sodas and sports drinks has exploded, as has the incidence of obesity, diabetes, hypertension, heart disease, cancer, and stroke. *Killer Colas* looks at the history and growth of the soft drink industry, explores its very powerful influence over the media, and examines the harmful ingredients that these companies include in their formulas. It also offers scientific evidence that links America's consumption of soft drinks with our declining health.

Killer Colas exposes the facts behind an addiction that is just as powerful and dangerous as our love of tobacco. Once you have read this book, you will never look at a soft drink in the same way.

$15.95 • 192 pages • 6 x 9-inch quality paperback • ISBN 978-0-7570-0341-7

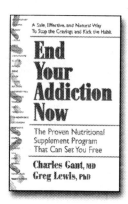

END YOUR ADDICTION NOW
The Proven Nutritional Supplement Program That Can Set You Free
Charles Gant, MD, and Greg Lewis, PhD

While a number of rehabilitation programs are available, too many people with addictions return to their old habits. *End Your Addiction Now* explores the biochemical factors that are the real cause of this problem and offers proven advice on how to break addictions once and for all. A distinctive program of nutritional supplements is designed to jump-start recovery, which begins with a natural process of detoxification. Biochemical testing pinpoints the specific deficiencies that must be addressed to achieve complete recovery.

$16.95 US • 304 pages • 6 x 9-inch quality paperback • ISBN 978-0-7570-0313-4

BIG YOGA
A Simple Guide for Bigger Bodies
Meera Patricia Kerr

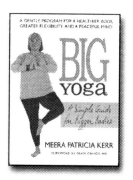

If you think yoga is only for skinny people, you need to think again. To expert Meera Patricia Kerr, yoga can and should be used by everyone—*especially* plus-size individuals. In her new book, *Big Yoga,* Meera shares the unique yoga program she developed for all those who think that yoga is not for them.

Part One of *Big Yoga* begins with a clear explanation of what yoga is, what benefits it offers, and how it can fit into anyone's life. Included is an important discussion of self-image. The book goes on to provide practical information regarding clothing, mats, and suitable environments, and to emphasize the need to begin with care. Part Two offers over forty different exercises specifically designed to work with bigger bodies. In each case, the author clearly explains the technique, details its advantages, and offers step-by-step instructions along with easy-to-follow photographs.

If you have thought that yoga is not for you, pick up *Big Yoga* and let Meera Patricia Kerr help you become more confident and relaxed than you may have ever thought possible.

$17.95 US • 240 pages • 6 x 9-inch quality paperback • ISBN 978-0-7570-0215-1